OVERCOMING BINGE EATING

Dr. Christopher G. Fairburn

THE GUILFORD PRESS
New York London

A Division of Guilford Publications, Inc.
72 Spring Street, New York, NY 10012

The information in this volume is not intended as a substitute for consultation with health care professionals. Each individual's health concerns should be evaluated by a qualified professional.

Printed in the United States of America

This book is printed on acid-free paper.

Last digit is print number: 9 8 7 6 5 4

Library of Congress Cataloging-in-Publication Data

Fairburn, Christopher G.
Overcoming binge eating / Christopher G. Fairburn.
p. cm.
Includes bibliographical references and index.
ISBN 0-89862-179-8 (pbk.) ISBN 0-89862-961-6 (hard)
1. Compulsive eating—Popular works. I. Title.
RC552.C65F35 1995
616.85'26—dc20 94-43152
CIP

Preface

If you have a binge eating problem (or you know someone who does), you probably have looked to a variety of sources for information on the subject. Chances are you ended up perplexed and discouraged, torn by conflicting opinions. Rather than gaining understanding and the means to overcome the problem, you may have ended up resigned to living with a problem that increasingly erodes your quality of life.

It doesn't have to be that way.

For many years I have been aware of the need for an accessible yet authoritative account of all aspects of binge eating. For nearly two decades I have been concentrating on developing and evaluating new treatments for these problems. This book is my answer to the need for a reliable source of information and the even greater need for a treatment program that works for a broad range of people.

Overcoming Binge Eating is organized to address two separate but interdependent goals: Part I presents the most current scientifically based facts about binge eating problems. Part II is a self-help manual founded on the most effective treatment for them.

If you binge, you may be tempted to go directly to the step-by-step instructions in Part II of the book, but I urge you to read Part I as well. Arming yourself with information empowers you to deal with your problem. But I also hope that once you possess the facts you will help spread the word. As this book demonstrates, an intricately woven web of misinformation not only prevents many people from stopping binge eating but has also led many to adopt this self-destructive behavior in the first place.

Recent media coverage has made most of us aware that binge eating is prevalent in Western society. It also has informed us that this potentially damaging behavior is a problem of young Caucasian women, that it is driven by "carbohydrate craving," that it is a pattern of eating caused by "yo-yo dieting." Unfortunately, none of these latter statements is true. All are, in fact, common misconceptions, and they are a mere sampling of the myths circulating today. Others are the extreme claims of some branches of the diet industry, which give people false hopes about the weight and shape they can possibly achieve. Failure to meet these unrealistic goals launches many people on a vicious circle of binge eating and dieting that can be difficult—but is not impossible—to break.

It is not only erroneous information that causes harm. Incomplete reports that omit important facts also promulgate unhealthy behavior. For example, there is evidence that people who attempt to control their weight by vomiting or misusing laxatives or diuretics commonly hear of these practices through the media. How many never would have adopted these practices if they had also heard about their adverse effects, let alone their ineffectiveness as means of weight control? Eating problems escalate once people begin "purging" along with bingeing; disseminating the truth about such behavior is one way of preventing serious problems from developing.

Part I of this book presents state-of-the-art knowledge in this field, a unique synthesis, unavailable elsewhere, of what is known about binge eating problems. Frequent trips abroad have given me the opportunity to learn from other clinicians' and researchers' experience as well as to share my own. As a result, this book represents a true distillation of current knowledge, not just my own impressions. Our understanding of binge eating is still far from complete, however. To ensure a balanced account, this book not only presents what we know but also points out what we do *not* know at this time.

The opening two chapters of Part I cover the fundamentals—how a true binge is distinguished from an episode of everyday overeating, the difference between binge eating problems and binge eating disorders, and the criteria clinicians use to diagnose the major forms of eating disorder. Whether you binge eat or know someone who does, it is important to understand exactly how this behavior is characterized. And if you do have a binge eating problem, Chapter 3 will assure you that you are far from alone; it offers all the data that the most current research studies have produced on who binges.

Chapters 4 and 5 delve more deeply into the nature of binge eating problems, describing the psychological, social, and physical problems associated with the behavior. Here you will find the facts about purging and other weight control methods—their ineffectiveness and the toll they can take on the body—and information on how bingeing and associated behaviors can affect other aspects of life.

The causes of binge eating are often difficult to identify. What we do know is that what causes a problem to develop and what keeps it going are not necessarily the same. Chapter 6 discusses the latest findings, and Chapter 7 addresses one issue that often arises in the United States in particular: Is binge eating a form of addiction?

Chapter 8 ends Part I by discussing the various approaches to treatment that have been used in the last twenty years, concluding that a specific psychological treatment called *cognitive-behavioral therapy* is clearly the most effective at producing *lasting* change. It is this treatment that underlies the self-help program in Part II.

Many people do not realize that the great majority of those with binge eating problems are not receiving any form of help. There are many reasons for this, as the book explains, one being that many people are reluctant to reveal their problem to anyone. This is one of the reasons that self-help programs have much to offer. Another reason is that the research on treatment suggests that self-help, alone or with minimal guidance ("guided self-help"), should be sufficient to help many people overcome their binge eating problem. The self-help treatment program in Part II can be used on your own or with the help of a therapist or trusted friend or relative, and it can also be applied in concert with other forms of treatment should this be necessary.

In my twenty years of work with those who have binge eating problems I have found that some people have little drive to change, or their drive wavers. They have come to accept their binge eating problem and adjust their life around it. In addition to seeking to educate and help, another goal of this book is to encourage people to change and make a fresh start. If you have a binge eating problem, I hope that this book stimulates you to tackle it; or, if you are doing so already, I hope it strengthens your resolve.

ACKNOWLEDGMENTS

It is a pleasure to acknowledge the many people who have helped me write this book. First and foremost I must thank Peter Cooper, a longstanding colleague and friend. Without his encouragement the book would never have been written. Peter has helped in many ways, not least by furnishing most of the illustrative quotations scattered throughout the text. He also provided insightful feedback on various versions of the manuscript. I also wish to thank those people with binge eating problems who have commented on the book and used the self-help program. Their contribution has been invaluable. In addition, I wish to thank those friends and colleagues who have read the manuscript and contributed to its evolution through successive drafts. I would particularly like to thank my wife, Susan, and colleagues Terry Wilson, Kelly Brownell, Marsha Marcus, Laura Hill, Jacqui Carter, Faith Barbour, Jenny Burton, Zafra Cooper, Beverley Davies, Valerie Dunn, Phillipa Hay, Pat Norman, Marianne O'Connor, Sue Shaw, and Christina Wood.

Finally, I would like to acknowledge Christine Benton and Seymour Weingarten. Chris, as editor, has added significantly to the book through her intelligent comments and insightful suggestions. Seymour, as editor-in-chief at The Guilford Press, has acted as a marvelous go-between. I am grateful to him for his support and encouragement and his commitment to the book.

Contents

PART I

BINGE EATING: THE FACTS

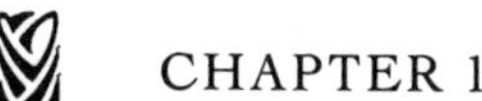

CHAPTER 1

What Is a Binge?

IT STARTS OFF with my thinking about the food that I deny myself when I am dieting. This soon changes into a strong desire to eat. First of all it is a relief and a comfort to eat, and I feel quite high. But then I can't stop, and I binge. I eat and eat frantically until I am absolutely full. Afterward I feel so guilty and angry with myself.

A generation ago the term *binge* meant one thing to most people: drinking to excess. Today the word more often means eating to excess. For many people a binge is something perfectly innocuous—a dietary slip or lapse, a simple overindulgence. For others, though, it signifies a loss of control over eating, and it is a major problem for a large number of people, notably young women in Western countries such as the United States and the United Kingdom.

Despite the fact that binge eating is undeniably widespread, a scientifically based understanding of it is not. Thanks in part to the distribution of much misinformation by the popular communications media, most people—those who have experienced binge eating and those who have not—know comparatively little about this problem.

Does everyone who binges also purge? Is binge eating a chronic condition, or can it be overcome? Is binge eating a passing aberration in the behavior of an otherwise "normal" person, or is it a sign that something else is wrong? What sort of person is likely to binge and why? When do binges occur, and what triggers them? How long does the typical binge last? How do we distinguish—in ourselves or those we care about—between a true binge and simple overeating? And often most important of all, how can people who binge stop this often destructive behavior?

None of these questions can be answered without a full understanding of what a binge is, and that is the goal of this opening chapter. What are binges like? When people binge, what do they eat and in what way? Are there different types of binge?

WHAT DOES *BINGE* MEAN?

As mentioned, the meaning of the word has changed over the years. In common usage since the mid–nineteenth century, *binge* then meant principally "a heavy drinking bout, hence a spree," according to the *Oxford English Dictionary*. While that remains one of its meanings, nowadays dictionaries often define a binge as overeating, and the term *indulgence* may be used. *Merriam Webster's Collegiate Dictionary*, Tenth Edition, for example, says one meaning is "an unrestrained and often excessive indulgence."

That so-called indulgence is an experience reported by at least one in five young women today. However, the significance of the experience varies considerably among them. Some view it as the occasional indiscretion mentioned earlier; it has no effect on their lives. For others, though—such as the woman whose description opened this chapter—it is a true problem, something that has a negative impact on many aspects of life.

Failure to understand that distinction—benign binge eating versus problem binge eating—is at the heart of much confusion about this behavior. Actually the misconceptions run even deeper: When should an episode of overeating be called a binge rather than everyday overeating? Recognizing the need to clarify these definitions, researchers have made intensive efforts to investigate the experiences of those who binge eat. While no two personal accounts are identical, it turns out that true binges have two features in common: The amount of food eaten is large, and there is a sense of loss of control at the time. The identification of this common thread has enabled the American Psychiatric Association to arrive at a generally agreed-on technical definition of the term *binge:*

> An episode of binge-eating is characterized by both of the following:
>
> (1) eating, in a discrete period of time (e.g., within any two-hour period), an amount of food that is definitely larger than most people would eat during a similar period of time and under similar circumstances, and,
>
> (2) a sense of lack of control over eating during the episode (e.g., a feeling that one cannot stop eating or control what or how much one is eating).

What is central to binge eating is the sense of loss of control. *This feature above all distinguishes binge eating from everyday overeating and mere indulgence.*

THE CHARACTERISTICS OF A BINGE

> *I randomly grab whatever food I can and push it into my mouth, sometimes not even chewing it. But I then start feeling guilty and frightened as my stomach begins to ache and my temperature rises. It is only when I feel really ill that I stop eating.*

Personal descriptions of binge eating can be tremendously revealing. For a variety of reasons, however, these accounts may not be fully accurate. Consequently some research groups have been studying binge eating in laboratory settings. One of the most sophisticated laboratories is the Pittsburgh Human Feeding Laboratory at the Western Psychiatric Institute and Clinic, University of

Pittsburgh (see box below). This laboratory is in fact unique, so the findings that it is just beginning to produce should prove invaluable to ongoing research.

Meanwhile, anecdotal information and the findings from other laboratories continue to add brushstrokes to the picture of a "typical" binge. What has emerged is a description that you might recognize, at least in part, if you binge or you think that someone you know binges.

Feelings. The first moments of a binge can be pleasurable. The taste and texture of the food may seem intensely enjoyable. Such feelings seldom last long, however. Soon they are replaced by feelings of disgust as the person consumes more and more food. Some people feel revulsion over what they are doing but are unable to stop.

Speed of Eating. Typically people eat rapidly during a binge. Researchers at Columbia University found that women with bulimia nervosa ate food more than twice as fast as women with no eating disorder: 81.5 calories per minute compared with 38.4 calories per minute. Many stuff food into their mouth almost mechanically, barely chewing it. Many also drink copiously to help wash the food down, and this contributes to their feeling full and bloated. It also helps some people vomit up the food afterward.

Agitation. Some people pace up and down or wander around during their binges. There may be an air of desperation about them. They feel the craving for food as a powerful force that drives them to eat. This is why the term compulsive eating is sometimes used (see Chapter 2 for another use of this term). Obtaining food takes on extreme importance; people may take food belonging to others, steal from stores, or eat discarded food. Most view such behavior as shameful, disgusting, and degrading.

I begin by having a bowl of cereal. I eat it really quickly and then immediately have two or three more bowls. By then I know that my

The Pittsburgh Human Feeding Laboratory

The Pittsburgh Human Feeding Laboratory, the only laboratory of its kind, is just beginning to produce findings as of the early 1990s. Its uniqueness lies in the fact that people can stay there for extended time periods—longer than 24 hours—while their behavior related to disturbed eating, such as self-induced vomiting, is measured.

The laboratory consists of a 19-square-meter room adjacent to an inpatient eating disorder treatment unit. It has a table, a chair and bed, and a television and videocassette recorder, and adjacent is a private bathroom. People are able to communicate with a control room by intercom.

Food is obtained from two computer-controlled vending machines, one of which is refrigerated. The food can be heated using a microwave oven. The vending machines contain 38 different types of food and drink chosen to represent those available in cafeterias and the type of food eaten in binges. The precise composition of all the food is known.

Over their stay of several days, people may be given various instructions. For example, they may be asked to binge or to eat what they would normally eat on a day when they do not binge. Both patients with bulimia nervosa and people with no eating problems have been studied. The people being studied are always made fully aware of what is involved, and their consent is obtained.

A laboratory of this type provides one means for obtaining detailed information on people's eating behavior. Although an obvious weakness is the laboratory's artificiality, there are reasons to think that people's behavior in the laboratory is similar to that outside because it often matches their prior accounts of their behavior. It is certainly clear that people with bulimia nervosa will binge in such a setting.

Source: Kaye WH, Weltzin TE, McKee M, McConaha C, Hansen D, Hsu LKG. Laboratory assessment of feeding behavior in bulimia nervosa and healthy women: Methods for developing a human-feeding laboratory. *American Journal of Clinical Nutrition* 1992; *55:* 372–380.

control is blown and that I am going to go all the way and binge. I still feel very tense, and I desperately search for food. These days this means running around college looking for food people have thrown out. I know that this is really disgusting. I stuff the food down quickly. Sometimes I go into town, stopping at stores along the way. I buy only a little from each store so as not to arouse suspicion. I stop when I have run out of money or, more usually, because I am so full that I physically cannot eat any more.

A Feeling of Altered Consciousness. People often describe feeling as if they are in a trance during a binge. If you have experienced this, you know that your behavior seems almost automatic, as if it is not really you who is eating. But people also report that they watch television, listen to loud music, or use some other form of distraction to prevent them from having to think about what they are doing.

It all starts with the way I feel when I wake up. If I am unhappy or someone has said something to upset me, I feel a strong urge to eat. When this urge comes, I feel hot and clammy. My mind goes blank, and I automatically move toward food. I eat really quickly, as if I'm afraid that by eating slowly I will have too much time to think about what I am doing. I eat standing up or walking around. I often eat watching television or reading a magazine. This is all to prevent me from thinking, because thinking would mean facing up to what I am doing.

Secretiveness. A marked characteristic of the typical binge is that it occurs in secret. Some people are so ashamed of their binge eating that they go to great lengths to hide it—and may succeed in doing so for many years. One way they accomplish this is by eating in a relatively normal manner when with others. Another is by exercising considerable subterfuge. Perhaps you are familiar with some of the ways that people report keeping their behavior hidden: After eating a normal meal, some people later return surreptitiously to eat all the leftovers. Others take food to the bedroom or bathroom to eat it without fear of detection.

I leave work and go shopping for food. I begin eating before I get home, but it is secret, with the food hidden in my pockets. Once I'm home, proper eating begins. I eat until my stomach hurts and I cannot eat any more. It is only at this point that I snap out of my trance and think about what I have done.

Loss of Control. As stated earlier, this is central to binge eating, but it varies considerably among individuals. Some people feel it long before they begin eating. For others it evolves gradually as they start to eat. Or it may come on suddenly as they realize that they have eaten too much.

Interestingly, some people who have been binge eating for many years report that their sense of loss of control has faded over time, sometimes because experience has taught them that their binges are inevitable and so they no longer try to resist them. Some even plan what they see as unavoidable binges, thus setting up a self-fulfilling prophecy. Planning allows these people to exercise some control over when and where their binges occur, thereby minimizing the disruption of their daily activities. They feel therefore that they have not in fact lost control. This is not really the case, however, since they are still unable to prevent their binges. Further, many report being unable to stop eating once they have started.

This seems to be the case even when a binge is interrupted. Food supplies may be exhausted, the telephone may ring, or someone may come to the door. When this happens, it is common for the binge to restart once the disruption ends. As Drs. Janet Polivy and Peter Herman of the University of Toronto have said, it is as if the binge eater is in "pause mode" at such times.

HOW AND WHEN PEOPLE BINGE

People vary widely in how often they binge and what foods they eat, so it is difficult to define a typical binge in these terms. Not surprisingly, how and when people binge continue to be the subjects of much research.

Frequency and Duration

To be given a diagnosis of the eating disorder bulimia nervosa (described in Chapter 2) according to the American Psychiatric Association's criteria, a person's binges have to occur on average at least twice a week. But this threshold of twice a week is arbitrary—a leftover of early attempts to define the disorder in the late 1970s—and thus has been criticized: it implies that people who binge less frequently are less disturbed when this is often not the case. Many researchers and clinicians believe that a threshold of once a week would be more appropriate. Consequently, clinicians treating people with eating disturbances often ignore arbitrary thresholds of this type when making a diagnosis.

The significance of frequency can also be confusing for the person who binges. If you binge "only once in a while," does this mean there is no need for concern? At what level of frequency *does* binge eating become a problem? Is it the numbers—how often you binge, for how long, over what time span, consuming how many calories—that determine how serious a problem exists? Or should the guiding factor be how much the bingeing affects your life? In practice clinicians are concerned with impairment—the degree to which the binge eating interferes with your physical health and general quality of life. There is no simple relationship between impairment of this type and the frequency of bingeing. In fact, in the early 1980s a study of forty patients with bulimia nervosa conducted at the University of Minnesota showed that many exceed the American Psychiatric Association's twice-a-week mark (see page 11), and more recent studies have confirmed this finding. On the other hand, it has also been shown that many otherwise typical patients binge less often than this.

How long do binges last? This depends on what kind of eating problem or disorder the person has. Current data from my research group in Oxford indicate that among those who purge afterward—those who compensate for their binges by inducing vomiting or misusing laxatives or diuretics—many binges last about an hour. But for those who do not purge, they last an average of almost twice as long. This is probably because those who purge feel pressure to complete their binges as soon as possible so that they can purge quickly, thereby minimizing the amount of food absorbed (see Chapter 4).

The Foods Eaten in a Binge

> *The food I eat usually consists of all my "forbidden" foods: chocolate, cake, cookies, jam, condensed milk, cereal, and improvised sweet food like raw cake mixture. Food that is easy to eat. Food that doesn't need any preparation. I never eat these kinds of food normal-*

Frequency and Duration of Binges in Patients with Bulimia Nervosa

In this study 40 patients with "bulimia" (the original American term for bulimia nervosa; see Chapter 2) kept daily records of the duration and frequency of their episodes of binge eating. These were the main findings:

1. The average duration of a binge was 78 minutes and ranged from 15 minutes to 8 hours.
2. The average number of binges was 11.7 over the one-week assessment period and ranged from 1 to 46 episodes. The most common pattern was to binge once a day, usually in the afternoon or evening.
3. The average number of calories consumed per binge was 3,415, ranging from 1,200 to 11,500 calories (data from 25 of the 40 patients).
4. The foods most commonly eaten were, in descending order of frequency, ice cream, bread, candy, doughnuts, salads, sandwiches, cookies, popcorn, cheese, and cereal.

Source: Mitchell JE, Pyle RL, Eckert ED. Frequency and duration of binge-eating episodes in patients with bulimia. *American Journal of Psychiatry* 1981; *138:* 835–836.

---

ly because they are so fattening. But when I binge I can't get enough of them.

When people who binge are asked "What do you eat when you binge?" they typically give two types of reply. The first relates to the character of the food. So they may reply, "sweet food" or "filling food." The second reply relates to their attitude toward the food. So they may answer, "forbidden food," "dangerous food," or "fattening food." What is clear is that most binges are composed of foods that the person is trying to avoid.

The Myth of "Carbohydrate Craving." You may have read that binges are characterized by their high carbohydrate content and are driven by a "carbohydrate craving"—a widespread myth. In fact, the proportion of carbohydrate in binges is not particularly high, no higher than that in ordinary meals. What characterizes binges is not their composition in terms of carbohydrate, fat, and protein, but rather the overall amount eaten. If you binge or know someone who does, you know that binges typically include cakes, cookies, chocolate, ice cream, and so on. But, as Dr. Timothy Walsh of Columbia University has pointed out, while it is commonly believed that these foods are high in carbohydrate, they are more accurately described as sweet foods with a high fat content. Dr. Walsh gives two examples: 57 percent of the calories in Haagen-Dazs vanilla ice cream come from fat, whereas only 36 percent come from carbohydrate; and even in devil's food cake 40 percent of the calories come from fat. Carbohydrate craving, although a popular notion and a memorable phrase, is a myth.

Interestingly, though, the term may have had more relevance some years ago. It is my impression that the composition of binges has changed over the last twenty years, with more carbohydrate-containing foods being consumed in the late seventies and early eighties. If so, this may reflect a change in dieting practices over the years: the focus was on excluding carbohydrates at that time, whereas these days fats are the target.

Figure 1 shows an eating record that includes a typical binge.

Day . *Wednesday* . . . . Date . . *April 8* . . . .

Time	Food and drink consumed	Place	*	V/L	Context and comments
8:15	(Weighed myself)				Can't write down my weight—it's gross.
8:50	Glass water	Kitchen			Thirsty after yesterday.
10:10	Diet coke	At work			Determined not to binge today.
11:30	10-20 Graham crackers Water	At work	*	V	Started by just eating a couple, and then, before I knew what I was doing, I was out of control.
12:05	Water				
6:50	Piece of apple pie ½ gallon ice cream 4 slices toast with peanut butter Diet pepsi 6 cupcakes 1 raisin bagel 2 pints ice cream Diet pepsi		* * * * * *	 V V	Started to eat as soon as I got home. Out of control immediately.
7:50	Two glasses water				Feel very lonely.
9:45	Glass water				Went to bed early.

Figure 1. An eating record showing a typical binge. (Asterisks signify eating viewed by the person as excessive. V/L signifies vomiting or laxative use.)

The Size and Cost of Binges

The amount of food eaten during binges varies widely from person to person. Some people consume vast quantities of food during a binge; occasionally a person describes eating 15,000 to 20,000 calories at one time. However, this is not typical. When people are asked to describe exactly what they have eaten and then the number of calories is calculated, the typical binge contains between 1,000 and 2,000 calories. About a quarter contain more than 2,000 calories—more than the average daily intake of many women. Significantly, laboratory studies have supported these accounts: Similar figures have been obtained when people have volunteered to binge and then the precise composition of their binges has been calculated. One recent study found that one in every five patients with bulimia nervosa had binges of more than 5,000 calories and one in ten had binges of more than 6,000 calories.

A significant finding of all these studies is that during some binges, which are otherwise typical, the person eats only average or even small amounts of food. These episodes do not meet the American Psychiatric Association's technical definition of a binge because of their small size, yet the person views them as binges because the characteristic sense of loss of control occurs. The Eating Disorder Examination, an interview for assessing the features of eating disorders, devised by the author and Dr. Zafra Cooper and considered the standard in the field, describes such binges as *subjective binges*. In contrast, binges in which truly large amounts are eaten are termed *objective* binges. A revealing fact about binge eating in general is that subjective binges are not uncommon and that they too can be a cause of considerable distress.

Not surprisingly, binge eating can be expensive. Those who regularly consume large quantities of food can get into financial difficulties. Figure 2 illustrates the cost of binge eating. It shows the cost of a single binge bought from a supermarket. In the early 1980s a study conducted in Chicago reported that the average cost of a binge was $8.30 with the range being between $1.00 and $55.00. The high cost of binge eating explains in part why some people resort to stealing food.

ARE ALL BINGES THE SAME?

Binges vary considerably not only from person to person but also within a single individual. Many people report that they have more than one type of binge, although some may not fit the technical definition of a binge (an objective binge). One person described having the following types of binge:

Full-Blown Binges

> *I eat and I eat, usually very fast, and without enjoyment, apart from initial taste-pleasure, which anyway is tempered with guilt. Usually furtively, and in one place—at home, the kitchen; at college, my room. I eat until I physically cannot eat any more. This is usually the type of binge where I take laxatives—during and after—which intensifies the feeling of panic and guilt. Immediately afterwards I*

THANK YOU
FOR SHOPPING
KEY FOOD

JIF CREAMY PNUT BUT	2.99
KEY COTTAGE CHEESE	1.39
DIET COKE 2 LITER	1.39
SINGLE SODA BOTTLE	.05
ARNOLD BRANOLA BREAD	2.29
HOSTESS BROWNIE BITE	2.99
HERSHEY CHOC KISSES	2.79
FAMOUS AMOS CH/CHP	2.99
HAAGEN DAZS	2.99
TOMBSTONE PIZZA	4.69
SLSTAX	.34
TOTAL	$24.90

10 ITEMS

Figure 2. The cost of binge eating. A supermarket receipt showing the cost (in U.S. dollars) of food bought for a single binge.

am so physically bloated that emotions are dulled, but later I feel terrible.

Half-Binges

These usually take place late at night and are similar to full-blown binges except that I eat food hurriedly in one place, and without enjoyment, but also without a great deal of panic. It is almost an automatic reaction, often to some situation. I can stop these.

Slow-Motion Binges

Usually I have these at home, not college. I can see them coming in advance. I may fight them for a while, but eventually I give in and have an almost pleasurable feeling. There's definitely a release of tension at the time because I don't have to worry anymore. I actually enjoy these binges, at least to start with. I choose foods that I like and don't usually allow myself or allow myself only in limited quantities. I may spend time preparing the food. At some stage it hits me what a fool I'm being and how much weight I will gain (not how greedy I am being), and then I become even more guilty, but I still feel a compulsion to carry on.

Certain groups of people have distinctive binges. For example, people with anorexia nervosa often have small, subjective binges, but with the same distress and sense of loss of control associated with objective binges. And the binges of people who are significantly overweight (many of whom have "binge eating disorder"; see Chapter 2) tend not to be clearcut in the sense that their beginning and end can be difficult to define. These binges generally last longer than those of people with bulimia nervosa; indeed, they can last almost all day. Also, the eating is slower and less desperate. Nevertheless, the amount of food eaten is truly large, given the circumstances, and there is a sense of loss of control at the time. The associated guilt and shame are also similar, as is the secrecy.

BEFORE AND AFTER: HOW BINGES BEGIN AND END

If you binge or you are trying to understand this disturbing behavior in someone else, you are probably baffled by the fact that it occurs at all. Why would something that leaves you feeling disgusted and ashamed happen again and again? What causes a binge eating problem to begin and what keeps it going are two broader issues, and they are addressed in Chapter 6. Also important, however, are the more immediate triggers of individual binges. What circumstances can make a binge begin?

Triggers of Binges

Many things trigger binges. In 1982 a study conducted in Australia produced a disparate list of triggers (see box below). Some of the most common triggers are described in the following paragraphs.

Unpleasant Feelings

> *Binges start when I'm tired or depressed or just upset. I become tense and panicky and feel very empty. I try to block out the urge to eat, but it just grows stronger and stronger. The only way I know to release these feelings is to binge. And binge eating does numb the upset feelings. It blots out whatever it was that was upsetting me. The trouble is that it is replaced with feeling stuffed and guilty and drained.*

Unpleasant feelings of all types may trigger binges. Feeling depressed is a particularly powerful stimulus. Other emotional triggers include tension, hopelessness, loneliness, boredom, irritability, and anger.

Feeling Fat. Feeling fat is a particular type of unpleasant mood that is common among people who are concerned about their shape (see Chapter 4). It can trigger binge eating.

The Triggers of Binges

In this study a detailed description was obtained of the binges of 32 patients seen at an eating disorder clinic in Sydney, Australia. These patients described 12 main precipitants of their binges.

91% tension
84% eating something (anything at all)
78% being alone
78% craving specific foods
75% thinking of food
72% going home (either after school or work, or after living away)
59% feeling bored and lonely
44% feeling hungry
44% drinking alcohol
25% going out with someone of the opposite sex
22% eating out
22% going to a party

Source: Abraham SF, Beumont PJV. How patients describe bulimia or binge eating. *Psychological Medicine* 1982; *12:* 625-635.

Gaining Weight. Most people who are concerned about their weight react badly to any increase. Any weight gain, even as little as a pound, may precipitate a negative reaction. Among those prone to binge, one response may be to abandon all attempts at controlling eating with the result being a binge.

Dieting and the Associated Hunger

The urge to binge usually begins around midday on a "normal" day—that is, a day on which I am trying not to eat. During the afternoon thoughts of food become more and more of a preoccupation; and eventually at around 4:00 P.M. my power of concentration will be sufficiently nonexistent for thoughts about food to be totally overwhelming. So I leave my work and go to the store.

One thing that definitely sets me off is hunger. If I am hungry, instead of eating something to satisfy it, I eat anything I can lay my hands on. It's almost as if I have to satisfy all tastes, even for things I don't like.

Many people with a binge eating problem eat little outside their binges. This food deprivation can have many undesirable effects, as it would for anyone who was essentially starving himself or herself. Eating too little results in physiological and psychological pressures to eat, and once eating starts those prone to binge can find it difficult to stop.

Breaking a Dietary Rule. Many people who binge also diet, and their dieting tends to be characteristic (see Chapter 4). For example, they often have strict rules about when and how much they should eat. In addition, they may have rules about what they should eat, with foods being banned if they are viewed as "fattening." Breaking a dietary rule commonly precipitates a binge.

Unstructured Time. Lack of structure in the day seems to make people prone to binge, whereas having a routine seems to be protective. Lack of structure may also be accompanied by feelings of boredom, one of the unpleasant moods that tends to trigger binges.

Being Alone. As already mentioned, binges almost always occur in secret. For those most prone to binge, being alone increases the risk since there are no social constraints against binge eating. If the person is lonely as well, the risk is even greater.

Premenstrual Tension. Some women report that they find it particularly difficult to control their eating in the few days before a menstrual period. This can be a response to physical sensations such as feeling bloated or negative moods such as depression and irritability.

Drinking Alcohol. Some people find that drinking alcohol makes them vulnerable to binges. There are a number of reasons for this. Alcohol reduces the ability to resist immediate desires and so interferes with adherence to dietary rules. For example, a plan to eat only a salad could, after a few drinks, be readily abandoned in favor of eating a full meal. Alcohol also impairs judgment and causes people to underestimate how bad they will feel if they break their dietary rules. In addition, alcohol makes some people feel depressed, thereby further increasing their risk of binge eating.

The Aftermath

> *After a binge I feel frightened and angry. Fear is a large part of what I feel. I am terrified about the weight I will gain. I also feel anger toward myself for allowing it to happen yet again. Binge eating makes me hate myself.*

After everyday overeating, most people either accept the episode as an indulgence ("naughty but nice") or have some feelings of guilt (really regret). They may decide to compensate by eating less and perhaps by getting some exercise, but their self-recrimination and compensatory behavior end there.

The aftermath of a binge is quite different. Those who binge may say they experience some immediate, though temporary, positive feelings. For example, they may feel a sense of relief. Feelings of hunger and deprivation will have disappeared, and perhaps the depression or anxiety that may have triggered the binge has been displaced. But these positive effects are soon replaced by feelings of shame, disgust, and guilt. Depression often sets in, with people feeling hopeless about ever being able to control their eating. Anxiety is also common as fears of weight gain take over. The negative feelings may be exacerbated by the physical aftereffects of binge eating, tiredness and stomach pains being particularly common. The fear of weight gain may be so intense that it drives some people to take extreme compensatory measures (described in Chapter 4). It is these compensatory behaviors that distinguish, in part, those who simply binge from those who have one of the eating disorders described in the next chapter.

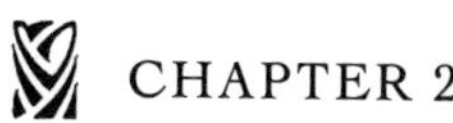

CHAPTER 2

Binge Eating, Eating Disorders, and Obesity

FEW PEOPLE TODAY are unaware that eating problems abound in the Western world. Most of us have heard of "bingeing and purging" and of the "slimmers' disease," anorexia nervosa; indeed terms related to binge eating have become such a part of the vernacular of popular culture that the term *anorectic* has become synonymous with *underweight.* In the process of working their way into the mainstream, unfortunately, the true meaning of many other terms describing disturbed eating has become blurred too. Popular magazine articles might bandy about terms like *eating problem* and *eating disorder,* using them interchangeably without regard to the distinction between the two. The truth is that *eating problem* does not mean "eating disorder" any more than *anorectic* means "extremely thin." What exactly is an eating problem, and when does it become an eating disorder?

The groundwork for answering this question was laid in Chapter 1, which discussed the difference between overeating and bingeing, a distinction that underpins the technical definition of a binge. This chapter follows up with a look at how psychiatrists and psychologists classify binge eating problems, how they are related to disorders, and where obesity fits in.

"EATING PROBLEMS" AND "EATING DISORDERS"

The great majority of people who binge have neither an eating problem nor an eating disorder. Their binge eating is occasional rather than frequent, it does not involve eating huge quantities of food, and it does not impair their quality of life. On the other hand, there are significant numbers of people whose binge eating does interfere, to a greater or lesser extent, with their quality of life. Their binge eating may be frequent, it may be distressing, and it may affect physical health. These people may be regarded as having an *eating problem*.

Many binge eating problems also fit the criteria for one of two *eating disorders,* bulimia nervosa or the recently described "binge eating disorder." If they do not, they still may resemble one of these two disorders. In a small minority of cases somewhat different eating problems exist. One of these is the eating disorder anorexia nervosa; other problems have not been defined well enough to be characterized clearly (see Figure 3). This chapter will describe what psychiatrists and psychologists mean by bulimia nervosa, binge eating disorder, and anorexia nervosa.

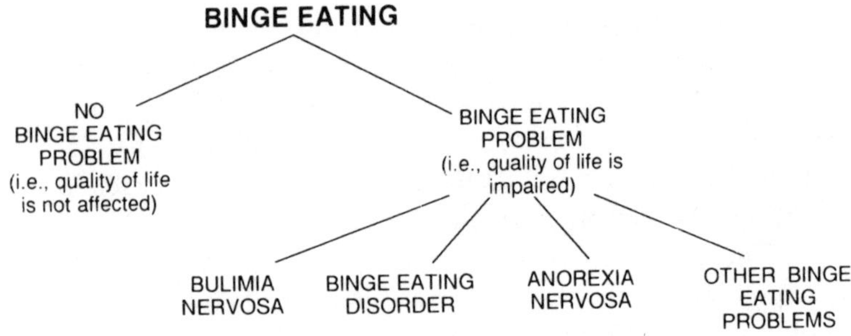

Figure 3. The classification of binge eating.

BULIMIA NERVOSA

Bulimia nervosa, originally known in North America simply as "bulimia," has come to medical attention only in the last twenty years. The box below lists the major milestones in the history of the disorder.

While modern diagnostic schemes differ in minor details, all agree that three things have to be present for someone to be said to have bulimia nervosa:

1. The person must have frequent (objective) binges; that is, he or she must consume genuinely large amounts of food, taking into account the context in which the food is eaten. The person must also have a sense of loss of control at the time.
2. The person must regularly use any one of a variety of ex-

A Brief History of Bulimia Nervosa

1976—Reports of "bulimarexia" among American college students (see Chapter 3).

1979—Publication of Professor Gerald Russell's classic paper "Bulimia nervosa: An ominous variant of anorexia nervosa." This paper provided the first description of the disorder.

1980—Syndrome of "bulimia" introduced into the American Psychiatric Association's *Diagnostic and Statistical Manual of Mental Disorders* (third edition).

1980–82—Studies in the United States and Britain indicate that bulimia nervosa is common (see Chapter 3).

1981–82—Reports describe two promising treatments, cognitive-behavioral therapy and antidepressant drugs (see Chapter 8).

1987—Syndrome "bulimia" redefined and renamed "bulimia nervosa" in the American Psychiatric Association's *Diagnostic and Statistical Manual of Mental Disorders* (third edition, revised) to bring it more in line with Russell's original concept.

---

treme measures for controlling shape or weight. These measures include self-induced vomiting, misusing laxatives or diuretics, overexercising, and intense dieting or fasting.

3. The person must be excessively concerned about his or her shape or weight or both (see Chapter 4) and should have an intense fear of fatness and weight gain. This concern should go beyond just feeling fat or being unhappy with his or her physical appearance. Rather, the person's whole life should be dominated by concern about body shape or weight.

Another requirement for the diagnosis is that the person does *not* fit the criteria for anorexia nervosa, a separate eating disorder described later in this chapter. In effect this means that the person cannot be significantly underweight. In practice the great majority of those with bulimia nervosa have a body weight in the normal range (defined as a body mass index between twenty and twenty-five; see Appendix I).

As explained in Chapter 3, bulimia nervosa is largely confined to women, most in their twenties. The problem usually starts in the late teenage years with a period of strict dieting. In about a third of cases this dieting may be so extreme that the person initially develops anorexia nervosa and then progresses to bulimia nervosa. So, while diagnostic rules stipulate that one cannot have the two disorders at the same time, they are obviously intimately related conditions.

People with bulimia nervosa have chaotic eating habits. By definition, all have objective binges. Typically their binge eating occurs in the context of extreme dietary restriction. Some eat virtually nothing between their binges, and the majority of the others diet strictly. Many make themselves vomit after each binge in an attempt to get rid of the food they have eaten. Laxatives or diuretics may also be taken for this purpose. Once established, this pattern of eating tends to be self-perpetuating, although it may wax and wane in severity. By the time people seek treatment, they often have eaten in this way for many years.

BINGE EATING DISORDER

Binge eating disorder is the other eating disorder in which binge eating is a central feature. It is a new diagnosis whose status is still somewhat controversial. Indeed many clinicians may not be familiar with the term, although many will be familiar with the problem it describes.

In the late 1950s Dr. Albert Stunkard of the University of Pennsylvania noted that some obese people had significant problems with binge eating. This observation was largely ignored or forgotten until the mid- to late 1980s, when evidence began to mount that about a quarter of those who seek treatment for obesity have binge eating problems, yet few fit the criteria for bulimia nervosa. At around the same time, community studies of the prevalence of bulimia nervosa showed that the majority of those who binge eat do not have bulimia nervosa (see Chapter 3). These findings led a research group headed by Dr. Robert Spitzer of Columbia University to propose that these people have their own eating disorder, one that is distinct from bulimia nervosa. They named the new disorder *pathological overeating syndrome,* since replaced by the less cumbersome *binge eating disorder.*

People with binge eating disorder have repeated binges, but they do not take the extreme weight control measures used by people with bulimia nervosa. Often in the past people who fit this description have been called—by professionals and nonprofessionals alike—*compulsive overeaters,* despite the fact that the term *compulsive eating* has no specific, recognized meaning. Clinical experience and research suggest that binge eating disorder has a broader distribution than bulimia nervosa. Men and women are more evenly affected; African-Americans appear to be at risk as much as Caucasians; and the age group seems to be broader, with people from twenty to fifty being affected.

It is a common misconception that *all* people with binge eating disorder are overweight. Community studies indicate that only about half are overweight (defined as having a body mass index of twenty-seven or more; see Appendix I).

ANOREXIA NERVOSA

Most people have heard of anorexia nervosa, the "slimmers' disease" (*slimmer* is a British term for "dieter"), perhaps because of a few widely publicized deaths associated with the disorder and because its physical effects are so obvious. Although it differs from bulimia nervosa and binge eating disorder in several important ways, it is, as said earlier, closely related to bulimia nervosa.

Two main conditions must be met for someone to be said to have anorexia nervosa:

1. The person should be significantly underweight, and this should be the result of his or her own efforts.*
2. The person should be highly concerned about his or her shape or weight or both. However, rather than worrying about being underweight, the person should be terrified of gaining weight and becoming fat. Indeed, many people with anorexia nervosa regard themselves as being "fat" despite their low weight. For this reason they are often said to have a "morbid fear of fatness" or a "weight phobia," and their dieting is said to be driven by a "relentless pursuit of thinness." These attitudes toward shape and weight are similar to those found in bulimia nervosa.

Anorexia nervosa mainly affects teenage girls and young women. People with the disorder achieve their low weight by eating very little, although excessive exercising may contribute. They avoid eating foods they view as fattening, and they may fast at times. About a third have "binges" during which their attempts to restrict their food intake break down and they lose control over eating. Dr. David Garner, a leading authority on anorexia nervosa, has pointed out that surprisingly little is known about the binges of people with anorexia nervosa. Clinical reports suggest

---

*What constitutes being significantly underweight? Definitions vary somewhat, but a person whose body mass index is below eighteen (see Appendix I) has an unusually low weight and is close to the threshold for anorexia nervosa.

that they are often small in size and thus would be considered subjective binges as defined in Chapter 1. Nevertheless, in other respects they are typical: There is a sense of loss of control over eating, and the amount consumed is *viewed* as excessive. For example, a binge may consist simply of a few cookies, but even this quantity of food will seem large to most people with anorexia nervosa. Irrespective of their size, the binges are associated with considerable distress and are followed by feelings of shame and guilt.

The classification and description of binge eating problems is an ongoing process. Future research is sure to shed light on forms of binge eating behavior not yet described in the scientific literature as well as to help us understand bulimia nervosa, binge eating disorder, and anorexia nervosa more fully. For now, though, the general definitions in this chapter should help you determine whether this diagnosis applies to you. If so, rest assured that you are not alone—as Chapter 3 reveals.

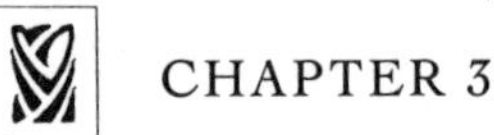

CHAPTER 3

Who Binges?

FOR ANYONE WHO BINGES, the question this chapter addresses can be the most compelling of all. Many people who binge, despite assurances to the contrary by the news media and others, feel alone in what they perceive as shameful behavior. That sense of isolation, unfortunately, perpetuates itself, preventing them from seeking help with the problem. So if you binge, the following pages may dispel that feeling of isolation, clearing a path toward recovery.

First, though, understand that those very feelings of shame and isolation and the resulting secrecy have made it difficult for researchers to find out exactly who binges. Because relatively few people seek treatment, pinpointing the incidence of binge eating is not as easy as counting the number of cases of measles or arthritis. Consequently, it is not absolutely clear how many people really binge rather than occasionally overeat. That caveat provided, this chapter will review what *is* known about who binges.

THE EMERGENCE OF BULIMIA NERVOSA

Interest in the number of people who binge originated with the emergence of bulimia nervosa in the mid-1970s. The first evidence of the disorder came with the publication of a number of reports describing "bulimarexia" or the "binge-purge syndrome" among female students on American college campuses. The disorder came to wider attention with the publication in 1979 of a paper titled "Bulimia nervosa: An ominous variant of anorexia nervosa" written by Professor Gerald Russell from London, a respected authority on anorexia nervosa. In this paper he described the characteristics of thirty patients (twenty-eight women and two men) whom he had seen over six and a half years between 1972 and 1978. These patients had bulimia nervosa as we know it today.

Simultaneously in Edinburgh, I was seeing a similar group of patients. The most striking thing about these patients was that the majority thought they were the only one with their type of eating problem. They thought that they alone had repeated bouts of uncontrolled overeating followed by vomiting or taking laxatives. This view was not surprising since bulimia nervosa had not yet attracted public attention. Indeed, in those days binge eating had hardly been heard of.

Most of my Edinburgh patients had successfully hidden their eating problem for many years. They had done this in part because of shame and self-disgust and in part because they thought that nothing could be done to help them. And keeping the problem hidden was not too difficult since most had an unremarkable body weight and most could eat relatively normally when with others. Their binge eating occurred in private. Some described summoning up the courage to see their family doctor, only to be told that they could not have an eating problem since their weight was normal.

The fact that bulimia nervosa could be kept hidden for many years meant that it might not, after all, be an unusual variant of anorexia nervosa as suggested by Professor Russell; rather, it might be a significant health problem in its own right. My problem was how to find out whether this was indeed the case. How could I uncover cases of this hidden eating disorder?

The solution was to enlist the assistance of the magazine *Cosmopolitan.* Since people with bulimia nervosa are highly concerned about their appearance, and since it seemed that most were young women, I guessed that many might read this magazine. So I arranged for a small notice to be placed in the April 1980 issue of the U.K. edition (see Figure 4). The result was dramatic. Within a few days I had received letters from more than a thousand women, the majority of whom seemed certain to have bulimia nervosa. This study is described in more detail on page 31.

More or less simultaneously in Chicago, Dr. Craig Johnson and colleagues were getting large numbers of requests for information following the publication of various popular articles on bulimia nervosa. They too sent out a number of questionnaires and in this way identified 361 women with bulimia nervosa (still termed *bulimia* in the United States at the time). These women were very similar to those identified through *Cosmopolitan,* although there were some curious and unexplained differences between the two samples, compared in Table 1.

New eating pattern

Some psychiatrists have become concerned recently over what may be the emergence of a new bizarre eating disorder affecting young women in their late teens and twenties. The principal features are frequent self-induced and secretive vomiting and a profound fear of becoming fat.

The sufferers have an irresistible desire to eat and drink, but keep their weight normal by vomiting.

The condition is difficult to treat—and many GPs may not be fully acquainted with the symptoms and dangers—but even in a mild form it can have serious physical and psychological repercussions.

Psychiatrists would like to know more about the prevalence of the disorder. Anyone with experience of vomiting this way might be able to help research by answering a confidential questionnaire.

Figure 4. The *Cosmopolitan* notice (from the Health Reports page of the April 1980 issue).

The *Cosmopolitan* Study

To find out whether bulimia nervosa was a significant, yet undetected, health problem, a notice was placed in the Health Reports page of the April 1980 issue of the women's magazine *Cosmopolitan* (see Figure 4). It requested people who were using self-induced vomiting as a means of weight control to write in if they were willing to complete a confidential questionnaire. Vomiting was chosen as the index feature for identifying potential cases of bulimia nervosa since it is the least ambiguous of the three core features of the disorder (see Chapter 2).

Within days more than a thousand replies were received. The first 800 were sent a questionnaire designed to obtain information on weight, eating habits, and attitudes toward shape and weight. Six hundred and sixty-nine questionnaires (84%) were returned fully completed. On the basis of the responses it was clear that 499 of the respondents were highly likely to have bulimia nervosa.

All 499 cases were women (remember, it was a women's magazine). Their average age was 24 years, and two-thirds were in their 20s. Over three-quarters (83%) had a body weight within the normal range for their age and height. In most cases the eating problem had started in their teenage years, and they had been binge eating, on average, for 5 years. A quarter (27%) reported that they were binge eating at least daily, and over half (56%) vomited daily. Nineteen percent abused laxatives.

The degree of distress reported by these women was extremely high. Many wrote lengthy letters pleading for help. Two-thirds (68%) had clinically significant levels of depressive and anxiety symptoms. Most expressed surprise and relief at knowing that they were not the only one with the problem.

Although over half these women thought that they definitely needed medical help, only 2.5% were receiving any form of treatment. Of those who wanted help, fewer than half (43%) had ever mentioned the problem to a doctor.

The findings of this study strongly suggested that bulimia nervosa was a significant, largely undetected, health problem.

Source: Fairburn CG, Cooper PJ. Self-induced vomiting and bulimia nervosa: An undetected problem. *British Medical Journal* 1982; *284:* 1153–1155.

At about the same time in New York, Dr. Katherine Halmi and colleagues of Cornell University were conducting a survey of binge eating problems among students attending a summer school. They found that over 10 percent reported significant binge eating problems, the great majority of whom were female, and almost 2 percent made themselves vomit at least once a week. In retrospect it seems likely that many had bulimia nervosa.

Since these studies were conducted, bulimia nervosa has been recognized as a significant health problem in a large number of countries, specifically those in which anorexia nervosa is encountered. It is now known to be common in North America, northern Europe, Australia, and New Zealand, and recently it has spread to Mediterranean countries such as Spain and Italy. It also

Table 1. A Comparison of the Samples Recruited in Two Early British and American Surveys of Bulimia Nervosa

	British sample	American sample
Age (in years)	23.8	23.7
Marital status		
Married (%)	20.7	18.4
Binge eating[a]		
Age at onset (years)	18.4	18.1
Duration (years)	5.2	5.4
Frequency—at least daily (%)	27.2	50.0
Self-induced vomiting		
Frequency—at least daily (%)	56.1	45.7
Laxative misuse		
Regular misuse (%)	18.8	33.0
Weight		
Normal weight[a]	83.2	61.6
Ever overweight (%)	45.2	50.1
Menstrual disturbance (%)	46.6	50.7

Sources: British sample—Fairburn CG, Cooper PJ. Self-induced vomiting and bulimia nervosa: An undetected problem. *British Medical Journal* 1982; *284:* 1153–1155.

American sample—Johnson CL Stuckey MK, Lewis LD, Schwartz DM. A survey of 509 cases of self-reported bulimia. In *Anorexia Nervosa: Recent Developments in Research.* Edited by PL Darby, PE Garfinkel, DM Garner, DV Coscina. Alan Liss, New York, 1983.

[a]Different definintions were used in the two studies.

appears to be emerging in central European countries such as the Czech Republic.

THE ISSUE OF DETECTION

The 1980 *Cosmopolitan* study found that only 2.5 percent of those identified as having bulimia nervosa were in treatment, a situation that has hardly changed since then. A recent British study, for example, found that out of fifty cases of severe bulimia nervosa, only six (12 percent) were receiving treatment, yet over half thought they needed professional help. A large study of psychiatric problems among teenagers in New Jersey got similar results: Few of those with bulimia nervosa had ever discussed their eating problems with a professional despite the fact that their day-to-day life was severely impaired. Indeed, it was found that bulimia nervosa was associated with the lowest rate of professional contact of all the problems studied (depression, panic, anxiety, and obsessive compulsive disorder). And there is evidence that binge eating disorder is also largely undetected.

Why are so few people with binge eating problems in treatment? There are many reasons:

1. These problems are accompanied by feelings of shame and guilt. By seeking treatment, sufferers run the risk of others finding out about their problem and the years of deceit and subterfuge that have been required to keep it secret.
2. People commonly hope the problem will go away on its own.
3. Some people think their eating problem is not severe enough to merit treatment or they do not deserve help.
4. There may be financial barriers to getting help. Sufferers may not have the financial resources or insurance needed to cover the cost of treatment.
5. It can be difficult to tell doctors. Previous medical problems (for example, menstrual problems; see Chapter 5) about which a doctor was consulted may have been a re-

sult of the eating problem, yet the doctor was kept in the dark about their true cause. Some people go to their doctor planning to divulge the problem but lose their nerve at the last moment.

6. Some doctors make it difficult to admit to problems of this type. For example, they may trivialize them.
7. Sometimes the doctor *is* told about the problem but does nothing about it; the doctor may not take the problem seriously, may not know what to do, or may not have access to suitable treatment facilities.
8. The doctor may provide help of an inappropriate nature. For example, some doctors simply hand out a diet sheet and do nothing else.

The fact that only a small proportion of those with binge eating problems are getting professional help creates a need for other sources of help, one of which is provided in Part II of this book. It also makes it difficult to answer the question "Who binges?" since hospital or clinic statistics grossly underestimate the magnitude of the problem. For this reason researchers have been studying community samples.

THE FINDINGS OF COMMUNITY STUDIES

Since 1980 more than sixty studies of the prevalence of bulimia nervosa have been conducted worldwide. Many have also produced figures on the prevalence of binge eating. The studies have focused mainly on women between the ages of fourteen and forty since they are thought to be most at risk. The majority have collected their data by asking people to fill out a number of simple questionnaires. One of their main findings has been that many young women report "binge eating." Indeed, across the studies over a third do so, and 16 percent report that they binge at least weekly. These are remarkably high figures. Can they be trusted?

For a number of reasons the reliability of these figures must be questioned. One reason is that most studies have not used the American Psychiatric Association's technical definition of a binge (see Chapter 1). Instead, many simply ask questions like "Do you binge?" and then take people's responses more or less at face value. As a result the figures are more likely to reflect those for any form of perceived overeating rather than true binge eating. Another problem is that over half of the studies have focused on female college students and often those enrolled at prestigious private universities. These students may not be representative of young women in general.

More reliable are the few studies in which general population samples have been interviewed. In most cases their goal has been to find out the prevalence of bulimia nervosa rather than that of binge eating. Interestingly, these studies have produced relatively consistent findings, indicating that bulimia nervosa affects between 1 and 2 percent of young adult women. With one exception, none of the studies has provided figures on the prevalence of binge eating as currently defined. The exception, a study from Oxfordshire in England, found that, among women aged sixteen to thirty-five, 10 percent had binges at least monthly and 3 percent had binges at least weekly. These figures are much lower than those obtained by the former group of studies, but they are likely to be more reliable since the assessment was done by interview and the new technical definition, not available at the time of the earlier studies, was used.

It seems therefore that about 1 percent of young adult women have bulimia nervosa and about 3 percent binge regularly. These figures are disturbing given that binge eating problems are often longstanding and can markedly impair quality of life (see Chapter 4), including physical health (see Chapter 5).

STUDIES OF OTHER DEMOGRAPHIC GROUPS

While community studies have given us a picture of the prevalence of bulimia nervosa among young adult women, it is becoming clear that neither this disorder nor binge eating disorder is restricted to this social group.

Older Women

The age distribution of bulimia nervosa strongly suggests that it is primarily a problem of younger rather than older women. As most studies have shown, the great majority of cases are in their twenties. Our community-based data from Oxford suggest that this may also be true of binge eating disorder although those who seek treatment appear to be on average somewhat older.

One of the few studies to have investigated older women found that, compared to younger women, few had *ever* had bulimia nervosa (see box below). This suggests that vulnerability to the disorder is a relatively recent phenomenon.

Men

Clinicians see few cases of bulimia nervosa among men, so it has seemed logical to conclude that the disorder is uncommon among them. Recently, however, claims have been made that the number of cases among men is increasing. Was the previous conclusion wrong? Perhaps men simply do not seek treatment or doctors do not detect the disorder or do not refer male patients for treatment. Neither explanation can account for the findings of the few general population studies to have included men. These studies, including the Christchurch study described on the opposite page and one that Dr. Peter Cooper and I did in conjunction with the British Broadcasting Corporation (see box on p. 38), have identified few cases. There is no foundation for the claims that the incidence of bulimia nervosa is increasing among men.

The prevalence of binge eating disorder among men is unknown. The results of a study published in 1991 suggest that it is distributed almost evenly between the sexes, but the reliability of this finding is questionable. The definition of binge eating used differed from today's technical definition, and the assessment was

The Christchurch Study

A general-population sample of adults aged 18 to 64 was recruited from the urban area of Christchurch, New Zealand. Of the 1,498 people interviewed, 994 were women with the following age distribution:

187: 18–24 years
590: 25–44 years
217: 45–64 years

The interview determined whether the person had *ever* had bulimia nervosa (lifetime prevalence). These were the results:

4.5%: 18–24 years
2.0%: 25–44 years
0.4%: 45–64 years

Since few of the older women reported having had bulimia nervosa in the past, vulnerability to the development of bulimia nervosa is apparently recent.

For the 504 men studied, much lower lifetime rates were obtained:

0.0%: 18–24 years
0.7%: 25–44 years
0.0%: 45–64 years

Source: Bushnell JA, Wells JE, Hornblow AR, Oakley-Browne MA, Joyce P. Prevalence of three bulimia syndromes in the general population. *Psychological Medicine* 1990; *20*: 671–680.

done by questionnaire rather than interview. In clinical samples of those with binge eating disorder, women far outnumber men.

Ethnic Group

Clinical experience suggests that bulimia nervosa occurs mostly among Caucasians. However, as noted elsewhere, data based on patient samples can be misleading. Recent North American sur-

The BBC Study

Following the publication of the *Cosmopolitan* notice in April 1980, the British Broadcating Corporation (BBC) made a television documentary on bulimia nervosa. This was broadcast in January 1981 and was the first time in Britain that bulimia nervosa received widespread publicity. The program described the problem in detail, and several sufferers (including one man) recounted their experiences. At the end of the program viewers were asked to write to the author if they thought that they had bulimia nervosa and were willing to fill in a confidential questionnaire. The response was overwhelming. Of the 1,827 questionnaires sent out, 1,391 (76%) were returned fully completed. From their replies 579 of the female respondents appeared highly likely to have bulimia nervosa.

There were also 45 male respondents, of whom two appeared to have anorexia nervosa and nine bulimia nervosa. The eating problems of these nine men closely resembled those of the 579 women.

These findings suggest that bulimia nervosa rarely occurs among men.

Source: Fairburn CG, Cooper PJ. Binge eating, self-induced vomiting and laxative abuse: A community study. *Psychological Medicine* 1984; *14*: 401–410.

veys suggest that binge eating disorder may be as common among African-American women as it is among Caucasian women.

People in Developing Countries

Very few studies have been conducted to discover the rates of binge eating problems among those in developing countries. They are thought to be rare.

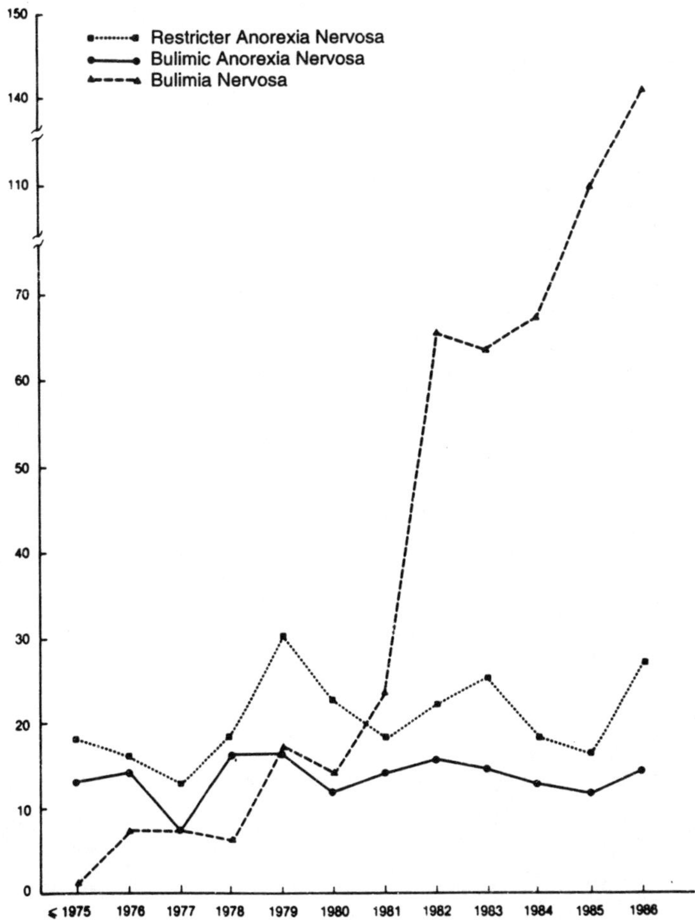

Figure 5. Rates of referral to a major eating disorder center in Toronto. *Source:* Garner, DM, Fairburn, CG. Relationship between anorexia nervosa and bulimia nervosa: Diagnostic implications. In *Diagnostic issues in Anorexia Nervosa and Bulimia Nervosa.* Edited by DM Garner, PE Garfinkel. Brunner/Mazel, New York, 1988. Copyright 1988 by Brunner/Mazel. Reprinted by permission.

CHAPTER 4

Psychological and Social Problems Associated with Binge Eating

SOMETIMES A BINGE IS JUST A BINGE. It is an isolated behavior that, even if recurrent, does not affect the quality of life. More often than not, though, binge eating is associated with other problems. You may, in fact, be reading this book because these problems are beginning to intrude on your health and happiness or those of someone you know. The relationship of such problems to the binge eating is often complex. Some problems are a true consequence of the binge eating; some are incidental associations of no particular significance; and some actually promote the binge eating. To make matters more confusing, some both stem from and encourage the binge eating—that is, they fall into both the cause and the effect sides of the equation. As such, they set off a vicious cycle that is difficult to break.

As this chapter will show, there is a circular element to binge eating that can make today's effect tomorrow's cause. So solving the entire web of problems is not always a straightforward matter of controlling the binge eating and then waiting for the other problems to disappear as an automatic consequence.

The goal of this chapter and the next is to describe all the problems and concerns associated with binge eating and to examine their possible roles in the eating problem. Understanding *how* they may be associated with binge eating, whether they are barely troublesome or major difficulties in their own right, can be crucial to arriving at the correct approach to treatment. This chapter looks at the problems that can be described as psychological and social; the physical problems are examined in Chapter 5. For more information on how these problems and others might cause binge eating, turn to Chapter 6.

DIETING

Most people who binge also diet. Dieting in fact is a good example of how problems associated with binge eating can defy classification as *either* cause *or* effect. Dieting often precedes binge eating in the development of binge eating problems, but it is also a response to overeating. As this chapter and Chapter 6 will show, there are good reasons to believe that dieting plays a key role in initiating *and* maintaining many binge eating problems.

Dieting interrupted by episodes of binge eating is a common pattern of eating. It is most obvious in bulimia nervosa and anorexia nervosa, where the dieting is generally extreme and persistent. Indeed, some people with these eating disorders eat little or nothing outside their binges. A similar pattern is followed by many of those with binge eating disorder, but the dieting is usually much less extreme, especially among those who are also overweight. Their dieting also tends to be intermittent rather than continuous. It is not uncommon for people with binge eating disorder to alternate between phases of successful dieting, which may last for months at a time, and periods of overeating. As a result, their body weight may fluctuate greatly.

Many people who have experienced some variation on this

type of eating pattern make the mistake of concluding that dieting is simply a response to binge eating. While it is undoubtedly encouraged by binge eating, especially among those who are highly concerned about their appearance and weight (discussed later in this chapter), the majority of people with binge eating problems were already dieting when they started to binge. And among those who diet strictly, the binge eating is *caused* at least in part by the dieting. As illustrated in Figure 6, there is a vicious circle, one that you may find familiar, with dieting both encouraging binge eating and being a response to it. The pattern can repeat itself almost indefinitely; it is a circle that can remain unbroken for years.

Because dieting is one of the main factors that makes people vulnerable to bingeing, reducing the tendency to diet is a goal of most treatments (see Chapter 8). If you wish to break a binge eating cycle or help someone else do so, you will find one way to achieve this in Part II of this book.

The Three Types of Dieting

There are three ways in which people diet, and people who binge—particularly those with bulimia nervosa—tend to practice all of them.

Avoiding Eating. Some people eat nothing at all between their binges. Indeed, they may not eat for days at a time (that is, they fast). More commonly, though, they avoid eating for as long

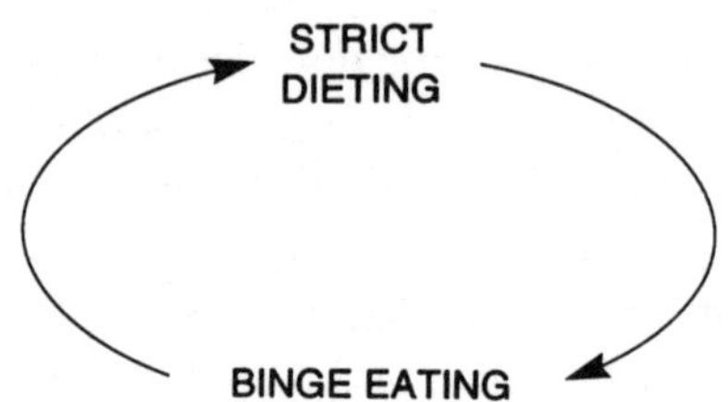

Figure 6. The cycle of dieting and binge eating.

as possible during the day, often not eating until evening. About one in four people with bulimia nervosa does this, though only about one in twenty with binge eating disorder does it. Among the general population, only about one in a hundred avoids eating all day.

Restricting the Overall Amount Eaten. Usually this approach involves trying to keep food intake below a specific calorie limit. For many people with bulimia nervosa the limit is set at 1,000 or 1,200 calories a day, well below the amount needed for normal day-to-day functioning. Some people set themselves even more extreme calorie limits. Liquid fast programs, for example, typically involve an intake of only 450 to 800 calories a day.

Avoiding Certain Types of Food. People who binge may avoid certain foods because they perceive them as fattening or because eating them has triggered binges in the past. They often describe such foods as "forbidden," "bad," or "dangerous." Research has shown that about one in five women in the general population diets in this way. In contrast, three-quarters of those with bulimia nervosa do so, as do half of those with binge eating disorder.

The range of foods avoided varies greatly. Among extreme dieters few foods—other than those manufactured and marketed as "diet foods"—are eaten freely. Figure 7 lists the foods avoided by one patient with bulimia nervosa.

Dieting in Other Guises. An interesting development is the adverse publicity that dieting has attracted recently, particularly in the United States. There antidieting campaigns have gone so far as to declare a "no dieting" day, and it is now unfashionable in some quarters to admit to dieting at all. As a result some people may describe their dieting as healthy eating or justify their restrictive eating practices on the grounds that they are vegetarians or have food allergies. However it is rationalized, any dietary restriction that is designed to influence shape or weight should be regarded as dieting.

Pasta
Pizza
Quiche
Tarts
Pies
Full fat cheese
Cake
pop
Chocolate
Honey
Jam and marmalade
Potato chips
Nuts
Eggs
Sandwiches
Mayonaise

Paté
yogurt
whole milk
Canned fruit
Ice cream
french fries
desserts
sweetened cereals
candy
butter
Cream
flour
Bread (some)
cookies

Figure 7. A list of foods avoided by a person with bulimia nervosa.

The Effects of Dieting

Food dominates my every waking minute. Even my dreams center on food.

The physical effects of dieting are described in Chapter 5. An important psychological effect is that the dieter becomes preoccupied with food and eating. Some people find themselves totally preoccupied with the very subject they are trying to avoid, unable to think about anything but food and eating. They find it difficult to engage in everyday activities requiring concentration, such as reading or conversing, and activities that demand minimal mental focus, such as watching television, become impossible. No matter what they are doing, thoughts about food and eating keep intruding into their mind. As Table 2 shows, such preoccupation is rare among young women in general, but as many as one in four of those with binge eating problems are affected to a moderate or marked degree. It's not hard to see how this preoccupation is likely to affect the ability to diet.

Strict versus Ordinary Dieting

The three types of dieting described so far are all *extreme;* that is the restrictions on how much, what, and when the dieter eats are severe. The dieting of some people who binge, particularly those with bulimia nervosa, also tends to be *strict.* Rather than having a general goal, these people have a very specific one, and if they do not achieve it they feel they have failed. Ordinary dieters might want to keep their calorie intake below, say, 1,500 calories a day and are likely to be content if they achieve this general goal on more days than not. In contrast, strict dieters feel that they *must* achieve this goal to the letter and that they have "failed" each time they eat more than their "rules" allow.

When dieting is both strict and extreme—involving highly specific dietary goals that demand considerable restraint—repeated "failures" are inevitable. This is demoralizing. To make matters worse, these failures tend to encourage binge eating. Typically, strict dieters who fail to meet a dietary goal give up temporarily and binge. Underpinning this reaction to the breaking of dietary rules is a thinking style characteristic of many of

Table 2. Preoccupation with Thoughts about Food and Eating among Women with Binge Eating Problems and Women in the General Population

	Women in the community (%)	Binge eating disorder (%)	Bulimia nervosa (%)
Little or none	95	57	49
Slight	3	18	23
Moderate	2	21	13
Marked	0	4	15

those who binge, so-called "all-or-nothing" or "dichotomous" thinking—described later in the chapter.

So, dieting governed by strict rules often perpetuates a cycle of binge eating and dieting, with each promoting the other. It is, however, important to understand that this vicious circle does not operate among all those who binge, just those who adopt strict dietary rules.

OVEREATING IN GENERAL

Interestingly, the overall eating behavior of people with binge eating disorder diverges somewhat from the diet-binge pattern just described. Those with bulimia nervosa fall into the all-or-nothing category of eating, while those with binge eating disorder also may overeat in general outside their individual binges. Research groups at the National Institutes of Health and Columbia University have found that people with binge eating disorder eat unusually large meals and also snack excessively. Thus it seems that in binge eating disorder there may be a general tendency to overeat as well as a specific vulnerability to binge eating.

OTHER MEASURES FOR CONTROLLING SHAPE OR WEIGHT

In addition to dieting, the weight control measure most commonly practiced by those with binge eating problems, some people adopt more extreme measures, including inducing vomiting and taking laxatives and diuretics. These forms of behavior are common in bulimia nervosa and anorexia nervosa but, by definition (see Chapter 2), rarely occur in binge eating disorder.

Self-Induced Vomiting

I had been anorexic for about a year and was attempting to start eating properly. One day, out of the blue, I ate a chocolate cookie. Suddenly I began eating all those things I'd deprived myself of. It wasn't a large binge by my current standards, but it was more calories than I normally ate in a whole week. I came out of my trancelike state and was suddenly terrified about what I had done. I immediately went to the bathroom and stuck my fingers down my throat. I had to throw up and get rid of all the garbage inside me.

I started vomiting after eating too much chocolate one day. It seemed a brilliant way to stay thin without dieting. I could eat as much as I wanted and then get rid of it. It would be so much easier than all that dieting.

It is not widely known that as many as 5 to 10 percent of young women admit to making themselves vomit, and as many as 2 percent of young adult women vomit as often as once or more a week. "Epidemics" of self-induced vomiting are sometimes reported, for example in some college dorms. As Table 3 shows, self-induced vomiting is common among people with bulimia nervosa, and it also occurs in up to half of those with anorexia nervosa. It is very much less common among those with binge eating disorder, and when it does occur it is occasional rather than frequent. While most of these people vomit to get rid of food they have eaten—that is, in an effort to limit the amount of food they will absorb—they may have other motives too. Tension release is the most common of these.

Self-induced vomiting is not necessarily evidence of an eating disorder as defined in Chapter 2. The key issue is whether the person has control over the behavior. For someone who chooses to do it on occasion, however socially unacceptable it might be,

Table 3. Common Methods of Weight Control (besides Dieting) in Bulimia Nervosa

	Community sample (%)	Clinic sample (%)
Self-induced vomiting	54	76
Laxative misuse	35	38
Both vomiting and laxative misuse	19	23
Diuretic misuse	10	12

the behavior is unlikely to be a sign of an eating disorder. But if the vomiting is frequent or cannot be resisted, it is almost certainly evidence of a significant eating problem.

Typically self-induced vomiting is achieved by sticking some object down to the back of the throat to induce the gag reflex. Often fingers are used, but some people use an implement such as a toothbrush. After a while some people can regurgitate at will by bending over and perhaps pressing on their stomach. There are others who cannot make themselves vomit, however hard they try.

> *I stop eating when I begin to feel ill. By then I have an overwhelming desire to rid myself of all the food I have eaten. I push my fingers down my throat and vomit again and again until I feel completely empty. This makes me feel relieved and cleansed. It also leaves me exhausted.*

> *I eat until I literally cannot eat any more. Then, using my fingers, I make myself sick. Over the next half hour, drinking water between vomits, I purge all the food from my stomach. I then feel despondent, depressed, alone, and desperately scared because I have lost control again. I feel physically terrible: exhausted, puffy-eyed, dizzy, weak, and my throat hurts. I am also scared because I know it is dangerous. After a couple of sessions of vomiting when I actually brought up blood, I tried to stop. But I continued to binge, and the fear that built up was so great that I started making myself sick again.*

Most people vomit after eating truly large amounts of food, but some people vomit after eating almost anything, particularly if they view it as fattening. Some people vomit just once after eating, and this rids them of sufficient food to relieve their anxiety over what they have eaten. Others vomit again and again until they cannot bring back anything more. This process can take an hour or more, and it leaves them physically drained. A minority practice a flushing technique: They drink something, then vomit, drink again and vomit, drink again, and so on, repeating this process until the liquid comes back clear of any food. Only at this point do they feel confident that they have retrieved everything that they can. This practice is dangerous (see Chapter 5).

You may have heard that some people eat "marker" foods (for example, tomatoes) at the beginning of binges and repeatedly vomit until these foods (the tomato skins) reappear in the vomit. Unfortunately, they are acting on the mistaken belief that what goes into the stomach first comes out last. Actually, the stomach contents are churned around, so the appearance of these markers does not necessarily mean the stomach has been emptied of everything eaten.

The belief that vomiting is an effective means of weight control is also somewhat false. While vomiting obviously gets rid of some of the food that has been eaten, a study of seventeen women with bulimia nervosa conducted at the Pittsburgh Human Feeding Laboratory (see Chapter 1) showed that self-induced vomiting resulted in the retrieval of less than half the food consumed during the average binge. The women, all of whom regularly vomited after binge eating, were asked to binge and vomit as if they were at home. When their calorie intake and the calorie content of their vomit was measured, the lab found that their binges averaged 2,131 calories and their vomit 979 calories. This explains why even those who vomit every time they eat are not necessarily underweight. They are living off the residue of their binges. How many of these people, you might wonder, would never begin self-induced vomiting if they knew that their body might still absorb over 50 percent of what was eaten?

> *I first started vomiting as a way of eating what I liked, without feeling guilty and without putting on weight. Vomiting was surprisingly easy and I was pretty pleased with myself. It was only later that I realized what a problem it had become.*

> *Over the past eight years I have repeatedly said to myself, "This is going to be the last time that I throw up." At first I was not that bothered: I thought I could control it if I chose to. But it soon became clear that it had control over me. Now stopping seems completely beyond my reach.*

Take a longer-term perspective, and the inadvisability of self-induced vomiting is even more obvious. People often describe the delight that they experienced when they discovered that they could make themselves sick. Here was the answer to their problems: Instead of struggling to control their urge to eat, they could give in yet not gain weight. In fact, for two main reasons they pay a heavy price. One is that vomiting encourages overeating. This is the result of two mechanisms. First, since people think that by vomiting they avoid absorbing what they have eaten, they tend to relax their controls over eating and eat more. Second, they discover that it is easier to vomit if their stomach is full. In this way a vicious circle gets established with the person becoming increasingly dependent on vomiting (see Figure 8). And the drive to vomit after eating can be extremely strong. Indeed, researchers from the University of Vermont have argued that in bulimia nervosa vomiting is one of the main factors that keeps binge eating going. They point out that many people with bulimia nervosa are able to resist binge eating if they know that they will have no opportunity to vomit.

Vomiting also has harmful physical effects. These are described in Chapter 5.

Laxative and Diuretic Misuse

I started taking laxatives because I was scared that because I was eating so much I would get fat really quickly. I thought that if I took laxatives all the food would go straight through me.

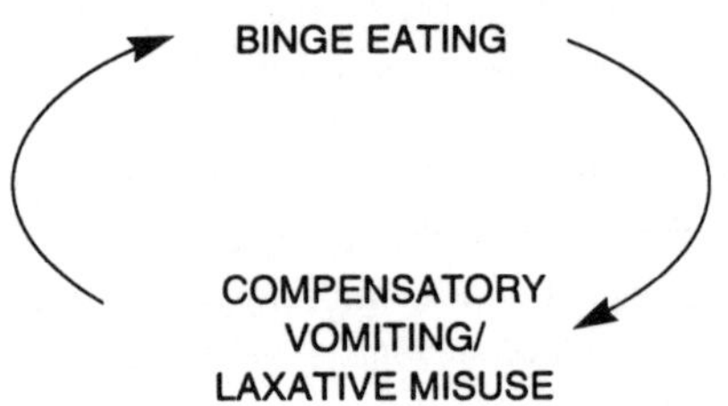

Figure 8. The cycle of binge eating, vomiting, and laxative misuse.

> *I read in a magazine about people using laxatives as a way of purging themselves. I'd tried vomiting but couldn't do it. So I went out and bought some laxatives and downed ten after every binge. I knew deep down that they didn't really do anything to counteract the binge, but they made me feel empty and cleansed inside.*

The use of laxatives or diuretics (water pills) to control weight is less common than self-induced vomiting. Laxatives are taken by about a third of those with bulimia nervosa and diuretics by about 10 percent (see Table 3). Both forms of misuse may occur in isolation or in combination with self-induced vomiting. All three forms of behavior are uncommon among those with binge eating disorder, although they do occur in anorexia nervosa.

People with binge eating problems misuse laxatives in two ways. They take them to compensate for specific episodes of overeating, in which case the behavior is very similar to self-induced vomiting and the numbers taken may be very large, or they take them on a regular basis, independent of particular episodes of overeating, in which casc the behavior is more like dieting. Diuretics tend to be taken in the latter way.

> *The hardest thing after a binge is waiting for the effects to die down. I hate feeling so useless and unable to do anything. Sometimes I feel I could literally rip open my stomach and pull out the garbage inside, the disgust and revulsion are so great. Failing that, laxatives are the next best thing.*

The physical effects of laxative and diuretic misuse are described in Chapter 5. Briefly, laxatives have little effect on calorie absorption, and diuretics have none. Nevertheless some people find the use of these drugs rewarding, mainly because there is weight loss, albeit transitory, due to the fluid lost in diarrhea or excess urine. In addition, some find that taking laxatives gives them a sense of having rid themselves, or "cleansed" themselves, of the food eaten. In this way laxatives, like self-induced vomiting, may encourage further binge eating. They may also like the feeling that their abdomen is empty, and some particularly like the flat appearance that may temporarily result. A minority also welcome the unpleasant physical effects. They see the abdominal cramps and spasms, and the associated diarrhea, as just punishment for having overeaten.

Diet Pills

Some people who binge take diet pills (appetite suppressants), bought by prescription or over the counter, in the hope of controlling their bingeing, despite the fact that there is no evidence that they have any effect on true binge eating.

Overexercising

Some people who binge exercise excessively to influence their shape or weight. As mentioned in Chapter 2, overexercising often contributes to the low weight of those with anorexia nervosa.

When those with a binge eating problem do overexercise, they do so in a driven or "compulsive" manner. They tend to spend an unusually great amount of time exercising and to make their exercise extremely strenuous. The other distinctive feature is that they have difficulty resisting exercising, even when the costs far outweigh the benefits. As a result, "overuse injuries" are not uncommon. When people with bulimia nervosa are asked why they exercise this way, it is often difficult to interpret their answer. Some acknowledge wanting to burn off fat or calories, but others do not, even though it seems that this is their main motivation. In extreme cases eating and exercising become so inextricably linked that people will not eat until they think that they have burned off the requisite number of calories in advance. This is termed *debting*.

In contrast, exercising too little is often a problem among overweight people with binge eating problems, many of whom have a sedentary lifestyle. This contributes both to their obesity and to its associated health risks. It therefore has to be addressed in treatment (see Appendix II).

CONCERNS ABOUT APPEARANCE AND WEIGHT

Most people who binge are highly concerned about their appearance and weight. Indeed, in those with bulimia nervosa these concerns are so intense that their life is dominated by them; nothing else is of such importance. Most want to lose weight, and almost all are terrified of weight gain.

Interestingly, however, these concerns do not necessarily predate the onset of the eating problem. Chapter 6 explains how the factors that cause binge eating problems to develop are not always the same as those that keep them going. Dieting has proved to be instrumental in both etiology (development) and maintenance, but at this point we are sure only that concerns about shape and weight tend to perpetuate existing binge eating problems by encouraging dieting.

> *My confidence and feelings of self-worth are deeply rooted in the idea that I must be physically attractive, i.e., thin. When I put on weight, even one pound, I risk being unattractive, and I see my future as bleak and lonely. This thought fills me with despair, so I force myself to eat as little as possible.*

Weighing becomes highly significant. Many go through periods during which they weigh themselves very frequently, in some cases many times a day. As shown in Figure 9, over one-fourth of those with bulimia nervosa weigh themselves at least once a day, compared to only one-twentieth of women in the community. Eventually, however, many people find weighing themselves so often intolerable. Consequently they switch to not weighing themselves at all. Even during periods when they are not weighing themselves at all, however, they remain highly concerned about their weight.

> *I am obsessed with my weight. I weigh myself over and over again, sometimes up to 15 times a day. At other times I am so disgusted*

with my body that I don't use the scales for weeks or months at a time.

Concerns about appearance are at least as common among those who binge as concerns about weight, if not more so. Despite the fact that there is no counterpart to the weighing scale, people adopt various methods for monitoring their appearance. They may regularly measure parts of their body, typically their thighs, or they may rely on the tightness of a certain piece of clothing.

Shame over how they think they look can interfere with day-to-day life. Many avoid letting others see their body. They may even avoid seeing it themselves. They might not be able to go swimming or to wear revealing summer clothes. Some people will not allow mirrors in the house. They may be unwilling to let their partner see them unclothed, and often their sex life is affected by their dislike of being touched where they view their body as fat. Telling these people that they look fine is rarely reassuring, as you may know; most are impervious to comments of this type or interpret them negatively.

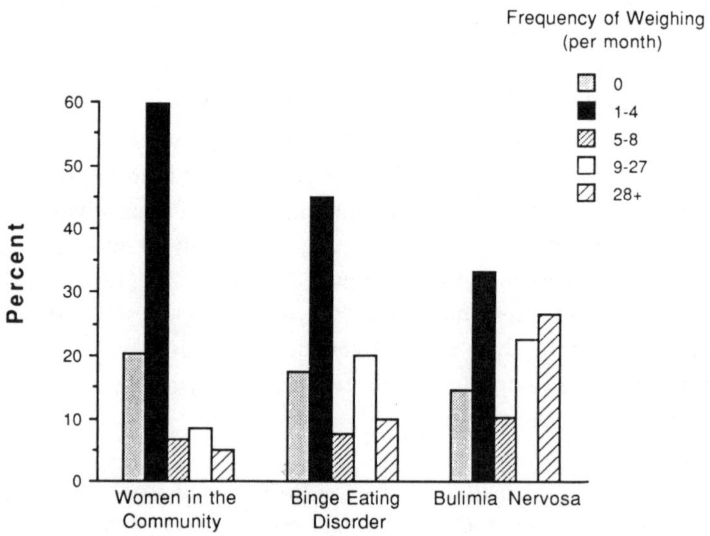

Figure 9. How often people weigh themselves.

I cannot put into words how repulsed I am with my body. I wish it were possible to wear clothes that disguised one's shape completely. I cannot bear to look at my body and will have no mirrors in the house. I take showers instead of baths to avoid having to look at myself. I have not gone shopping for clothes for more than three years.

I am confident in many ways, yet I hate my body and can't bear to look at it. I feel bloated, wobbly, and huge all over. This drives me to binge. My boyfriend loves me. Why can't I like myself?

If you've observed or experienced these concerns about appearance and weight, you know that they go above and beyond what researchers at Yale University have termed the "normative discontent" (the level of concern among women in the community) of many women today. For example, about one in ten women reports "feeling fat" at least daily, compared to over half of those with bulimia nervosa. The extreme nature of these concerns is even more striking when juxtaposed against the normal weight range of the majority of those with bulimia nervosa (see Chapter 5). And, as you're aware if you've known someone with anorexia nervosa, it is still more striking when the person is severely underweight.

People with binge eating disorder, particularly those who are overweight, are also concerned about their appearance and weight. This is hardly surprising given the social pressures to be slim. However, their concerns tend to have a different quality from those of people with bulimia nervosa; they are somewhat more understandable in view of their weight, and they are less extreme. Nevertheless, they are a problem. For example, like those with bulimia nervosa, many obese people who binge go to great lengths to prevent others from seeing their body, and they may also avoid seeing it themselves. Some view their body with disgust and loathing.

Still, concern about appearance and weight has particular significance in bulimia nervosa and anorexia nervosa. It is central to the maintenance of these disorders; it drives the dieting, vomiting, and misuse of laxatives and diuretics discussed earlier. And it is exacerbated by the episodes of loss of control over eating (see Figure

10 and Chapter 6). Reducing the intensity of these concerns is therefore a major goal of treatment (see Chapter 8 and Part II).

EFFECTS ON MOOD AND RELATIONSHIPS

> *My eating problem has taken over my whole life. My friendships have been upset by my violent swings in mood. I never talk to my parents since they have never understood what I am going through, yet we were so close. I have so little self-confidence. I get terribly depressed and anxious. I can't face seeing people.*

> *My life revolves around my eating. I can no longer concentrate on my work, which has suffered as a result. My problem has caused family rows. I no longer enjoy sharing meals with family or friends. I have become withdrawn and introspective and have lost all self-confidence and self-respect. I don't want to go out. I don't like myself anymore.*

As you are aware if you have a binge eating problem, particularly bulimia nervosa, quality of life suffers. You may feel depressed

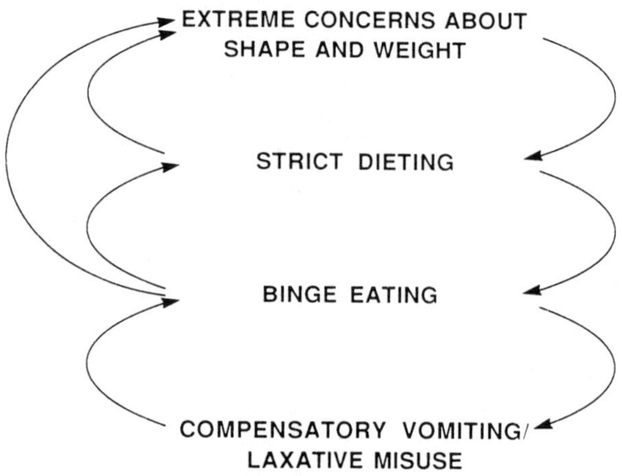

Figure 10. The central role of concerns about shape and weight.

and demoralized. Many people are ashamed of their lack of willpower and feel guilty about their secrecy and deceit. They are highly self-critical. Some get so desperate that they attempt to take their life. In most cases the depression, although severe, seems to be secondary to the eating problem; it usually lifts once the individual regains control over eating. Feelings of worthlessness may remain, however; in such cases there is often evidence of longstanding low self-esteem. In a minority, perhaps one in ten, the depression does not seem to be secondary to the eating problem. In these cases treatment directed at the depression may be required.

Those who binge are also prone to be anxious, and some avoid social occasions, especially those that involve eating. This might mean missing the wedding of a close friend, the graduation party of a favorite cousin, a birthday party of a parent—all of which hurt both the person with the eating problem and friends or family. In addition to anxieties of this type, mood swings are common, and some people are irritable and prone to outbursts of anger. A small number even injure themselves, sometimes as a means of releasing tension. Alcohol and drug problems may also be present (see Chapter 7).

At their worst, binge eating problems affect every aspect of life. Nothing is spared. So much time and effort is taken up by the problem that little is left for anything else. Relationships with family and friends may even become unsustainable.

Childrearing may also be impaired. Though at present our knowledge about the effects of binge eating problems on childrearing is based solely on cases in which difficulties have occurred, there is evidence that some people with bulimia nervosa dislike the chubby appearance of their baby and try to slim him or her down. Some limit the amount of food in the house to reduce their risk of binge eating or stock only diet food. Both practices restrict the food available for their children. And when children are older, daughters in particular may be put under pressure to join their mother on diets. It is not hard to see how this might put them at risk of developing an eating problem of their own (see Chapter 6).

As with feelings of depression, many interpersonal problems improve markedly, if not go away altogether, when the binge eating problem recedes. One of the most gratifying aspects of helping people overcome binge eating problems is seeing the person underneath gradually emerge as the problem goes away. The depression, tension, and irritability fade, concentration improves, and old interests return.

PERSONALITY CHARACTERISTICS

Binge eating problems disguise people's true personalities. Nonetheless, certain character traits are common among those who binge, and often they were evident well before the eating problem began.

Low Self-Esteem

Feelings of inadequacy and worthlessness are common among those with binge eating problems. While they are often part of the accompanying demoralization and depression, and so improve as the eating problem is resolved, they can also be the expression of a longstanding personality trait. Some people describe such feelings stretching back into their childhood.

Perfectionism

Another common longstanding characteristic is perfectionism; many who binge tend to set unduly demanding standards for themselves. Their perfectionism tends to affect all aspects of their life, but it is particularly obvious in the dietary goals that they set for themselves. This trait does, of course, have its positive side: Perfectionists may perform exceptionally well at, for example, work and sports. The key issue is whether their standards are realistic. If not, then these people will experience repeated "failures" even when their performance is high by most standards. Failing in this way can be undermining, especially if self-esteem is already low. Indeed, the combination of low self-esteem and perfectionism is especially common among those who binge and probably contributes to the development of the problem (see Chapter 6).

All-or-Nothing Thinking

All-or-nothing thinking (dichotomous thinking) is also common among those who binge. They tend to view things in extreme black or white terms. For example, they may class days as either good or bad; feel either in control or out of control; view foods as either dangerous or safe. This thinking style tends to permeate all thinking and not just that concerning eating. It is often associated with perfectionism. So, for instance, people who binge may define success in any contest or examination as coming in first; anything else is failure.

All-or-nothing thinking encourages binge eating since it leads people to abandon control after the slightest dietary transgression. It also leads them to set strict, highly specific dietary goals rather than general dietary guidelines.

Impulsivity

As will be discussed in Chapter 7, a minority of people with binge eating problems have problems with alcohol or drugs. Clinicians have noted that some also have other problems with impulse control. For example, they may be somewhat promiscuous or they may have a gambling problem. Professor Hubert Lacey of St. George's Hospital in London has suggested that these people have a "multi-impulsive" disorder and that their binge eating is just one expression of it.

Table 4 shows data from my research group on the rates of impulse control problems among women with binge eating problems, women with mood disorders, and women in the general population. All the women were recruited directly from the community. It is clear from these data that such problems affect only a minority of those in the two binge eating groups, the most prob-

Table 4. Impulse Control Problems in Women with Binge Eating Problems, Women with Mood Disorders, and Women in the General Population

	Women in the community (%)[a]	Binge eating disorder (%)[b]	Bulimia nervosa (%)[c]	Mood disorders (%)[d]
Problems controlling:				
Drinking alcohol	2	14	10	2
Using illegal drugs	0	0	1	0
Smoking cigarettes	6	25	23	12
Nail biting	13	31	21	18
Sexual behavior	0	2	6	2
Gambling	0	0	1	0

[a]Total = 100 [b]Total = 49 [c]Total = 100 [d]Total = 50.

lematic behaviors being smoking and nail biting. Nevertheless, Professor Lacey is certainly correct in stating that some people with binge eating problems do have general difficulties with impulse control. Since these behaviors often seem to be used to release tension, their treatment should include the development of skills for dealing with stress in less harmful ways.

Borderline Personality Disorder

A suggestion that overlaps with the idea of a multi-impulsive disorder is that "borderline personality disorder" is common among those with binge eating problems. The features of borderline personality disorder are listed in Table 5. There are at least two problems with this suggestion. The first is that the whole notion of borderline personality disorder is controversial. The second is that certain features of borderline personality disorder may appear in some people as a *result* of the eating problem. This view is supported by the observation that these features often disappear once the eating problem has resolved. If they were a sign of underlying personality disturbance, they would still be evident.

Table 5. The Features of Borderline Personality Disorder

Note: Not all features may be present in a single individual.

Unstable and intense relationships
e.g., alternating idealization and devaluation; fears of abandonment

Identity disturbance
e.g., poor sense of self; disturbed self-image; feelings of emptiness

Mood disturbance
e.g., intense and rapidly fluctuating mood states

Impulsive behavior
e.g., excessive spending, sex, or substance use; reckless driving; binge eating; lack of control of anger

Recurrent threatened or actual self-harm
e.g., suicidal threats or behavior; self-mutilation

Source: Adapted from the American Psychiatric Association, *Diagnostic and Statistical Manual of Mental Disorders* (fourth ed.). American Psychiatric Association, Washington DC, 1994. Copyright 1994 by the American Psychiatric Association. Adapted by permission.

Nevertheless, some people do seem to have many of these features. Research conducted at the University of Chicago and more recently at Stanford suggests that such people need more treatment than others with binge eating problems.

PREGNANCY

I am very anxious not to go over 140 pounds as I know it is going to be hard to lose all the weight. I hope to breast-feed, which I expect will help. Since I've stopped work I have been able to do lots of exercise. I swim thirty laps about five times a week, weight train twice a week, and I cycle about five miles most evenings. I also do Jane Fonda workouts.

I try to control my eating but find it difficult. After making myself vomit I feel extremely guilty as I would never forgive myself if any harm came to my baby - but I am pleased that I have stopped taking laxatives.

I worry about my eating problem affecting my relationship with my baby and my ability to cope. I hope to have three children, but I don't like the idea of getting pregnant again. Maybe next time I won't still be bulimic.

I had done really well with my eating. I had stopped vomiting and taking laxatives the moment I found out I was pregnant. I had also stopped binge eating. And I was trying really hard to eat only healthy foods. And then I was examined by my doctor and, when he was feeling my tummy, he looked up at me and said, "I am sorry I am taking so long, but I can't tell which is the baby and which is you." I know he was just joking, but it really upset me. I went home and cried. I ate nothing at all for the next few days, and when, with my husband's help, I did start eating again, I found that I could no longer resist vomiting afterward.

The great majority of those who binge are women of childbearing age. Despite this, little is known about the effects of binge eating on pregnancy. (See Chapter 5 for an account of the physical effects.) The work to date has tended to focus on those with bulimia nervosa. The pregnancies of those with binge eating disorder have yet to be studied.

The work on bulimia nervosa suggests that binge eating problems generally improve once the women knows that she is pregnant. The desire not to harm the fetus is strong, and for some it is sufficiently powerful to prevent them from bingeing altogether during pregnancy. The rate of self-induced vomiting also tends to decline, and most people stop misusing laxatives. Interestingly, dietary cravings occur just as in other people's pregnancies. These cravings can lead to the consumption of foods that would otherwise be avoided (such as ice cream), and, as a result, they may trigger binges.

Although I really wanted to control my eating, it was very difficult as my body seemed to take over in certain ways. I had cravings for foods that I would never normally eat. I found that I had to submit to them from time to time, which made me feel extremely guilty.

While pregnant many women with binge eating problems experience some degree of reprieve from their concerns about their appearance and weight. They feel that they are no longer accountable for them: Changes in their appearance and weight are inevitable. As a result, some give up their attempts to control their food intake and overeat instead. This puts them at risk of excessive weight gain, which, in turn, increases the risk of pregnancy complications. It also means that there will be more weight to lose following the birth.

> *As my pregnancy progressed, I still tried to control what I ate, calorie counting all the time and trying to keep under 1,500 calories a day. I also exercised every day. I still had regular binges although deep down I didn't want to cause any harm to my baby. I even had a binge the day that my labor pains began.*

On the other hand a minority of women with binge eating problems remain just as concerned about their appearance and weight, if not more so. The prospect of the change in shape and increase in weight terrifies them, and they fight it. They may diet, and some exercise heavily, sometimes as a substitute for vomiting or taking laxatives. As a result, they gain little or no weight, and at birth their babies may be underweight.

> *It is now three months since I gave birth. I've never felt so exhausted. I try to go for a run three to four times a week and I do lots of stomach exercises. I'd like to lose 15 pounds to get back into my prepregnant clothes. So far, my attempts at dieting have failed. My eating was very controlled when I first came home, but gradually the binges have returned and they are once again part of my daily life.*

Following childbirth everything changes. Many women find that any improvement in their binge eating problem was temporary and that it returns with a vengeance. This is not altogether surprising since many are determined to get back to their original weight as quickly as possible and therefore resume strict dieting almost immediately. This is their downfall since, as discussed earlier, strict dieting makes people prone to binge. And dieting is particularly difficult at this time. Many will be breast-feeding and so subject to increased physiological pressures to eat, and almost all will find their old routines disrupted.

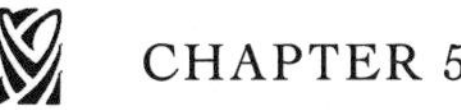

CHAPTER 5

Physical Problems Associated with Binge Eating

BINGE EATING PROBLEMS are associated with a diverse range of psychological and social difficulties. Over time they can transform an ordinary, happy existence into a miserable one, harming not only the person with the problem but also relationships with family and friends. Chapter 4 may have helped you understand the confusing behavior of someone you know and how it could be connected with a binge eating problem. Or it may have highlighted how your own life has been affected. Certainly it should now be obvious that binge eating is not innocuous behavior, and this chapter shows that its effects are not only psychological. Binge eating can damage the body in many ways, usually either as a direct result of the overeating or as a consequence of associated weight control behavior such as dieting and vomiting. Many of the physical effects of binge eating are reversible, but some are permanent. Most become worse with time, so they should not be ignored.

THE PHYSICAL EFFECTS OF BINGE EATING

Effects on the Stomach

I stop eating when it is impossible for me to continue—when I am literally full. After a binge I feel so full that my stomach hurts and I can hardly move. I feel sick, and sometimes, when I have had a particularly bad binge, even breathing is difficult and painful.

Binge eating has few immediate physical effects. Most objective binges leave the person feeling full, and in some cases the feeling is intense and painful. As Table 6 shows, people with bulimia nervosa are more likely to feel extremely full after a binge than people with binge eating disorder. This probably reflects the relative speed of eating.

People who eat until they are very full sometimes describe becoming breathless. This is caused by the distended stomach pressing up on the diaphragm. Very rarely, the stomach wall becomes so stretched that it is damaged or even tears. This is a serious medical emergency. If you develop abdominal pain when bingeing, it is essential that you stop eating. And if the pain is extreme, get help immediately.

Table 6. How Full People Get after Binge Eating

Bulimia nervosa
- 7%—do not feel full
- 7%—feel slightly uncomfortable (bloated, definite physical sense of having overeaten)
- 60%—feel moderately uncomfortable (distended but no pain)
- 26%—physically impossible to continue eating due to painful severe distension

Binge eating disorder
- 17%—do not feel full
- 32%—feel slightly uncomfortable (bloated, definite physical sense of having overeaten)
- 47%—feel moderately uncomfortable (distended but no pain)
- 4%—physically impossible to continue eating due to painful severe

Obesity

The relationship between binge eating and obesity is not simple; indeed, it is complex and far from fully understood. While few people with bulimia nervosa are overweight, obesity is common among those with binge eating disorder. This distinguishing characteristic has been mentioned in earlier chapters, and Figure 11 shows in detail how the two groups differ in terms of body mass index, a measurement of weight (explained fully in Appendix I). It seems natural to conclude that this distinction stems from the fact that people with bulimia nervosa take extreme weight control measures such as self-induced vomiting and misuse of laxatives while those with binge eating disorder tend not to do so. But for several reasons, the relationship between obesity and binge eating is not that simple. Does binge eating cause obesity, or does obesity cause binge eating? Or is some other mechanism at work? Let's look at some of the possible relationships.

First, it would be logical to predict that binge eating would make people obese or at the very least gain weight (path 1).

Path 1:

Binge eating → Obesity

Again, the prevalence of obesity among those with binge eating disorder seems to bear out this cause-and-effect relationship. On the other hand, it has been established beyond doubt that body shape and weight are strongly determined by genetic factors. So it could be that people with binge eating problems are genetically programmed to be overweight and that this leads them to diet, which in turn results in their starting to binge (through the mechanisms discussed in Chapter 4). In other words, rather than the binge eating leading to obesity, the reverse could be the case: Obesity results in binge eating (path 2).

Path 2:

Obesity → Dieting → Binge eating

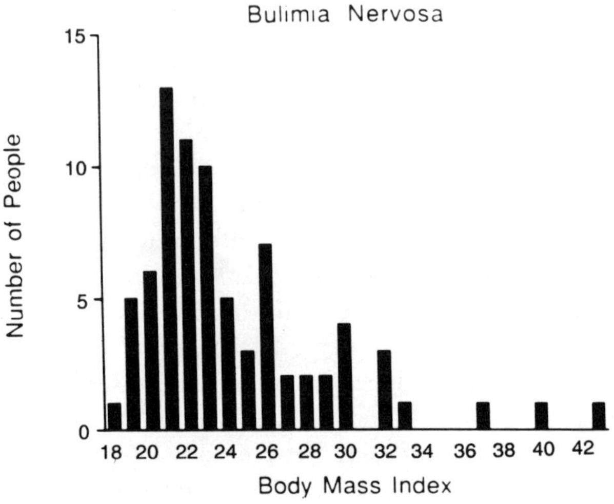

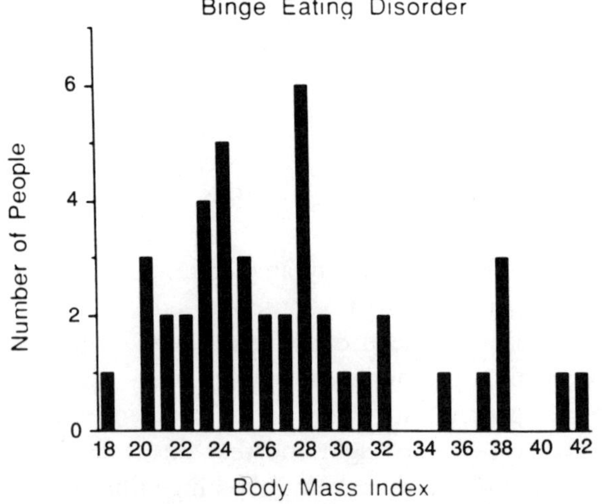

Figure 11. Body weight measurements for people with bulimia nervosa and binge eating disorder. A "body mass index" above 27 indicates a person is overweight. Healthy body weight is between 20 and 25.

The only reliable way to find out whether binge eating causes obesity or vice versa is to track how people change over time to discover which comes first, and this has yet to be done. Certainly one of the ways that binge eating problems develop may be via obesity. But even when obesity precedes the binge eating (path 2), it seems likely that the binge eating, once begun, will contribute directly to maintaining or worsening the obesity, thereby setting up a vicious circle (path 3). For this reason, and as explained in Part II, people with binge eating problems who are overweight may expect to lose some weight if they stop binge eating, although the weight loss may be slow and not as great as they would like.

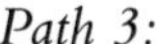

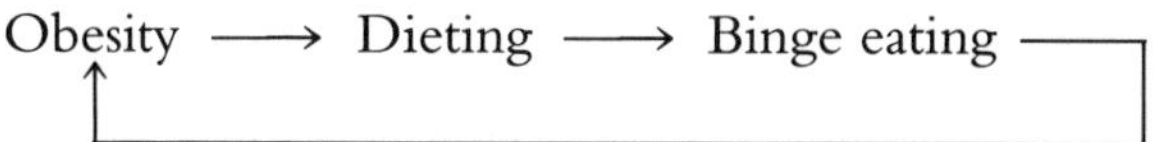

How are obesity and binge eating related in specific eating disorders? We already know that many people with binge eating disorder tend to overeat in general as well as binge (see Chapter 4), and this of course affects their weight. Because they overeat outside of their binges, they are unlikely to lose much weight once they stop binge eating unless the treatment of their binge eating also addresses their general tendency to overeat (see Part II).

What about people with bulimia nervosa? What happens to their weight with treatment? As mentioned earlier and shown in Figure 11, the great majority start treatment with a weight in the normal range. Some experts have argued, however, that while their weight may be normal statistically speaking, they are in fact below their "natural weight." In other words, they are presupposing that people with bulimia nervosa are naturally heavy. They support this view with the evidence that there is a higher-than-expected rate of obesity in these people's families and that some were themselves overweight before they developed the disorder. If this view were correct, those who make a full recovery—with a complete normalization of eating habits, including ceasing to diet—should gain weight. We have, however, found that this is not the case. For example, the findings of a recent treatment study conducted by my group in Oxford indicated that those who were fully recovered had on average virtually no change in weight between starting treatment and follow-up sixteen months later: These patients' average weight was 137 pounds before treatment and 134 pounds sixteen months later. However, these figures do reflect only the average. As Figure 12 shows, some patients lost much more weight than this and some gained. In the final analysis, though, these figures provide no grounds for saying that the weight of people with bulimia nervosa is naturally high.

Apparently a complex relationship exists between obesity and binge eating problems. In binge eating disorder, any weight problem is likely to be maintained by the binge eating and general tendency to overeat. In bulimia nervosa, while vulnerability to obesity may put people at increased risk of developing the disorder, true obesity is rarely a problem—rather, the key problem is the *fear* of obesity. As discussed in Chapters 4 and 6, this fear appears to play a central role in the perpetuation of the disorder.

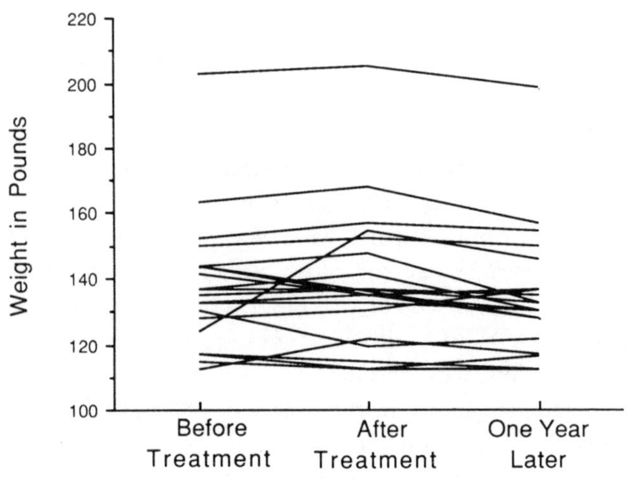

Figure 12. Change in weight on recovery from bulima nervosa.

PHYSICAL EFFECTS OF DIETING

Besides the psychological effects described in Chapter 4, dieting can have adverse physical effects. For example, it has been suggested that repeated cycles of weight loss and regain (weight cycling)—sometimes called "yo-yo dieting," a term that implies that the weight cycles are due to the individuals repeatedly going on and off diets—may alter body composition and metabolism in ways that make subsequent attempts to lose weight more difficult. Recent research suggests that this does not happen, although Dr. Kelly Brownell and colleagues have obtained evidence that weight cycling (or weight variability) is associated with a raised mortality rate, in particular an increased risk of death from cardiovascular disease. Why this should be so is not clear.

Dieting and weight loss can also affect body hormones, resulting in irregular or absent menstruation. Because regular menstruation requires a certain minimum level of body fat (see box below), women with anorexia nervosa do not menstruate. But even when body fat is adequate, dieting can affect menstruation,

Could Mannequins Menstruate?

At least 17% of their body weight must be fat for women to begin menstruating at puberty, and at least 22% must be fat for them to have regular menstrual cycles.

Investigators from Helsinki, Finland, measured the height and various other dimensions of mannequins from the 1920s on. They calculated their percentage of body fat as if they had been real women. Before the 1950s, they found, the amount of fat was mostly in the normal range. Thereafter, it was considerably less. They concluded that a woman with the shape of a modern mannequin would be unlikely to menstruate.

Source: Rintala M, Mustajoki P. Could mannequins menstruate? *British Medical Journal* 1992; *305:* 1575–1576.

though the underlying mechanism is unknown. This hormonal disturbance is seen in up to half of those with bulimia nervosa and about one in four of those with binge eating disorder.

In addition, dieting disturbs certain of the physiological mechanisms that control eating. It is now known that the nutritional composition of food (particularly the amount of carbohydrate, fat, and protein) has an important influence on the mechanisms controlling appetite. For example, one normal effect of eating carbohydrates is a potent and rapid suppression of hunger. A person who avoids carbohydrate-containing foods is thus denying herself that natural appetite suppressant. Interestingly, dieting has been shown to affect certain chemical transmitters in the brain, particularly serotonin, and this effect is more pronounced in women than in men. Since serotonin is thought to play a role in the normal control of eating as well as in food selection, this finding is intriguing. It also provides a possible physiological basis for the observation that a family or personal history of depression increases the risk of subsequently developing bulimia nervosa (see Chapter 6), since abnormal brain serotonin function is implicated in the etiology of depression. Put simply, it seems that an abnormality in brain serotonin function may put people at risk of developing bulimia nervosa and that dieting in women may exaggerate this risk.

PHYSICAL EFFECTS OF SELF-INDUCED VOMITING

As discussed in Chapter 4, self-induced vomiting is common in bulimia nervosa. It also occurs in anorexia nervosa, particularly among those who binge. It is practiced by about one in ten overweight people who binge, but the vomiting is occasional rather than regular.

Not surprisingly, repeated self-induced vomiting has a number of adverse physical effects, seen most often among those who vomit frequently and have done so for some time. As explained here, some of these effects are potentially serious.

Damage to the Teeth. Repeated vomiting over a long period of time damages the teeth, gradually eroding the dental enamel mainly on the inner surface of the front teeth. Dental fillings are not affected, so they become prominent relative to the surface of the enamel. Dentists can readily identify this characteristic pattern of erosion and may therefore deduce its cause. The erosion of the enamel is irreversible but not progressive—in other words, it stops once the vomiting stops. The practice of rinsing the mouth with water after vomiting is thought to accelerate the dental erosion rather than retard it.

Swelling of the Salivary Glands. Surrounding the mouth are glands that produce saliva. In some people who induce vomiting these glands gradually swell. This swelling is painless, but it may increase the production of saliva. Often it is the parotid gland (the gland commonly affected in mumps) that swells most, giving the face a somewhat rounded, chubby appearance. People with parotid swelling tend to see their face as "fat" and assume that the rest of their body looks the same. Naturally this increases their concern about shape and weight, thereby perpetuating the eating problem.

The swelling of the salivary glands is reversible and gradually goes away as eating habits improve.

Damage to the Throat. As described in Chapter 4, most people induce vomiting by mechanically stimulating the gag reflex. This can be a difficult and long process requiring force. Superficial injuries to the back of the throat sometimes result, and these may get infected. Complaints of recurrent sore throats and hoarseness are not uncommon.

Damage to the Esophagus. Very rarely, violent vomiting results in the tearing and bleeding of the wall of the esophagus, the tube that leads from the mouth to the stomach. There is a remote risk of rupture of the esophagus. This is a medical emergency. The presence of significant amounts of fresh blood in the vomitus should be taken very seriously and medical advice sought. It may come from an injury to the esophagus.

Damage to the Hands. One other mechanical effect of self-induced vomiting is seen in some people who use their fingers to stimulate the gag reflex. It is damage to the skin over the knuckles of the hand used. Initially abrasions appear on that hand, and eventually scars form, a highly characteristic abnormality known in medical textbooks as "Russell's sign" because it was first described by Professor Gerald Russell from London in his classic paper on bulimia nervosa.

Electrolyte Imbalance. The physiological effects of frequent vomiting can be serious, particularly among those who attempt to "wash out" their stomach by repeatedly drinking and vomiting until there is no sign of food in what they are bringing up. The balance of body fluids and electrolytes (sodium, potassium, etc.) can be disturbed in a number of different ways, some of which are serious. The electrolyte disturbance of most concern is hypokalaemia (low potassium) since it can result in heartbeat irregularities.

The symptoms of fluid or electrolyte disturbance can include extreme thirst, dizziness, fluid retention leading to swelling of the legs and arms, weakness and lethargy, muscle twitches and spasms. However, despite the fact that up to half of those with bulimia nervosa prove to have fluid and electrolyte abnormalities of some sort, most have none of these symptoms, and the electrolyte disturbance is mild. It is also important to note that all these symptoms can have other causes. So their presence is not necessarily indicative of an underlying electrolyte abnormality.

Such electrolyte disturbances are reversible and promptly go away once vomiting stops. Rarely do they require treatment in their own right, and any treatment should be supervised by a physician. For example, you should not take potassium supplements without regular blood checks.

A small number of people induce vomiting chemically. For example, they may drink salt water to make themselves sick. This is particularly inadvisable since it is another cause of electrolyte disturbance. Others take the over-the-counter drug Ipecac (ipecacuanha) to induce vomiting—a dangerous practice because several toxic effects result from long-term use.

PHYSICAL EFFECTS OF LAXATIVE MISUSE

As explained in Chapter 4, people who binge may take laxatives to influence their shape and weight, though the practice is less common than self-induced vomiting and is pursued mainly by people with bulimia nervosa. Some people take very large quantities, as many as 50 or a 100 at a time. Regardless of the amount taken, laxatives have little effect on calorie absorption. They act on the lower part of the gut, whereas calories are absorbed higher up. What they do produce is watery diarrhea and a temporary fall in weight due solely to the loss of water. The person regains the lost weight almost immediately as the body rehydrates. Nevertheless, people with bulimia nervosa find the weight loss rewarding, believing that it is evidence of an effect on calorie absorption, which is the main reason they persist in taking laxatives. As with self-induced vomiting, one wonders how many people would never begin misusing laxatives if they knew how ineffective they are.

Laxative misuse, like self-induced vomiting, produces a variety of fluid and electrolyte abnormalities with symptoms of the type just described. Individuals who both vomit and misuse laxatives are at particular risk. Some laxatives, when taken in high doses over long periods, result in permanent damage to the gut wall. Generally, however, the adverse physical effects are reversible. Someone who has taken laxatives regularly may retain fluid (water) for a week or so after stopping suddenly. Obviously this will produce a temporary weight gain.

PHYSICAL EFFECTS OF DIURETIC MISUSE

Some people take diuretics (water tablets), usually over-the-counter preparations, to change their shape and weight. Again, this is a fruitless exercise since diuretics have no effect on calorie absorption. Like laxatives, they cause fluid loss, in this case through the production of excess urine, and thus have a short-lived effect on body weight. When taken in large quantities, they can produce fluid and electrolyte disturbance. This is reversible. And, as with laxatives, those who stop taking diuretics after having used them for some time may experience temporary fluid retention. Clearly, they should not take further diuretics at this point, or they will establish a vicious circle.

EFFECTS ON FERTILITY AND PREGNANCY

To date little research has been done on the effects of binge eating problems on fertility and pregnancy. We know that dieting and weight loss impair fertility, an effect that is generally reversible (see box below). The influence of binge eating on its own has not been studied.

Binge eating is unlikely to affect the course or outcome of pregnancy, although when it is associated with obesity the risk of complications such as high blood pressure increases. More harm-

Dieting as a Cause of Infertility

Some women with unexplained infertility are strict dieters. Often they are underweight. When 29 such women were referred to a weight-gain program, 26 of them ended up gaining enough weight to be near their ideal. Nineteen of these women (73%) subsequently conceived spontaneously. Three would not accept the idea that dieting might be responsible for their infertility. None of these women returned for further care.

Source: Bates GW, Bates SR, Whitworth NS. Reproductive failure in women who practice weight control. *Fertility and Sterility* 1982; *37*: 373–378.

ful are likely to be the weight control behaviors of extreme dieting, vomiting, and the misuse of laxatives or diuretics. It is well established that during pregnancy those with anorexia nervosa are at risk of gaining too little weight and may give birth to underweight babies, and the same may be true of some mothers with bulimia nervosa. The findings of a study done by researchers at the University of Minnesota suggest that among women with bulimia nervosa the miscarriage rate may be increased. This finding, however, requires confirmation.

CHAPTER 6

Causes of Binge Eating Problems

I BEGAN BINGE EATING when I was about seventeen. I was lonely, shy and lacking in self-esteem. Every binge made me feel worse, made me hate myself more. I punished myself with more and more food. Within months I was binge eating as a matter of course and I gained weight rapidly. I loathed myself and continued with ordinary life only by pretending to be "normal."

Circumstances improved, and I binged less. However, my eating habits remained atrocious. Food was always on my mind. I never admitted my problems to anyone. And I lied to myself—denying what I had eaten or that I had eaten at all. Now, looking back on it all, I think of the years (almost sixteen) wasted, thinking about food and how fat I am. So many years spent depressed and hating myself.

Stories like this one raise an obvious question: Why did this binge eating problem develop, and why did it persist? As we've stressed throughout this book, not all binge eating problems are this severe or last this long. But anyone who has ever felt the distress accompanying loss of control over eating has probably asked, "Why?"

Unfortunately, there is no simple—or complete—answer. Our understanding of the cause of binge eating problems is still limited. One thing is clear, however: No single factor is responsible. We have already, in fact, looked at a diverse array of psychological, social, and physical factors that might be causes as well as effects of binge eating (see Chapters 4 and 5). In this chapter we'll delve more deeply into these factors and others. Certainly not all of them will pertain to everyone, but an overview of what we know can provide a valuable perspective on an individual's problem and may suggest appropriate treatment.

WHY THE CAUSES ARE SO ELUSIVE

As Chapter 8 and Part II will make clear, rarely can binge eating problems be resolved overnight. Expecting to pinpoint the cause and eradicate it—or advocating the sort of abstinence promulgated by some twelve-step programs (see Chapter 7)—is unrealistic. So, before you become dismayed by how often what we do *not* know is pointed out in this chapter, it might help to understand why the causes of binge eating are so difficult to unravel. It should also be heartening to know that, while the causes of these problems are ill understood, much more is known about how best to treat them (see Chapter 8).

Many Different Factors Are Involved

Social, psychological, and physical factors all seem to play a part in causing binge eating problems. Chapter 3 mentioned, for example, that bulimia nervosa has emerged only recently and only in certain countries. This suggests that environmental factors play a role in causing the disorder. Because environmental factors such as infectious agents can be ruled out, the recent emergence of bulimia nervosa can probably be attributed to social factors. We have also seen some of the psychological factors that come into play, such as the low self-esteem and perfectionism described in Chapter 4. And, as this chapter will show, genetically inherited factors also appear to contribute, which means that physical factors play a role too.

Several Routes Can Lead to Binge Eating Problems

The little research that has been done on the development of binge eating problems suggests that there is more than one route to these problems. There are at least four likely pathways.

Pathway 1. As mentioned earlier in this book, it is well established that bulimia nervosa is often preceded by anorexia nervosa, which, in turn, is commonly preceded by dieting:

Dieting → Anorexia nervosa → Binge eating → Bulimia nervosa

Typically the person begins dieting and losing weight in the mid-teenage years, despite in many cases not having been overweight in the first place. When the weight loss is extreme, it leads to the development of anorexia nervosa. Eventually, after a varying amount of time, the person's control over eating starts to break down and he or she begins to binge. Control progressively deteriorates, and the person's weight gradually returns to near its original level.

Pathway 2. A very different pathway is described by many people with binge eating disorder, particularly those who are overweight. They report having had a weight problem in their childhood, well before they began binge eating. For them, the progression seems to be from obesity to dieting and from dieting to binge eating:

Obesity → Dieting → Binge eating

As opposed to pathway 1, these people seem to begin dieting in response to obesity of varying degrees.

Pathway 3. Others with binge eating disorder describe having overeaten from an early age, dieting in response to the overeating, and the dieting only making matters worse—they continued overeating and at the same time developed a sense of loss of control:

Overeating in childhood → Dieting → Binge eating

Exactly when in this sequence weight problems develop, if indeed they do, seems to vary from person to person.

Neither pathway 2 nor pathway 3 involves a stage when the person is significantly underweight, although at times substantial amounts of weight may be lost as a result of dieting.

Pathway 4. The fourth pathway to binge eating is probably less common than the other three. It is direct and not via dieting. It is seen most often among those with a number of impulse control problems (see Chapters 4 and 7). With such people, the use of the impulsive behavior to release tension seems to be a key factor. Dieting does not appear to play a significant role.

Although these four pathways are the most common ones reported, it is important to realize that others occur and that some people follow a combination of them.

The Course of Binge Eating Problems Varies over Time

The third reason why determining the causes of binge eating is so difficult is that the outcome varies from individual to individual. For some, the problem is short-lived and will not recur. For others, recurrences and relapses will take place. For still others, once the problem begins it will stay with them for many years. This can only mean that additional factors, often separate from those that are responsible for starting the problem, come into play to keep it going.

What governs whether a binge eating problem persists or remits is not altogether clear. We've already pointed out in Chapter 4 that strict dieting, all-or-nothing thinking, and low self-esteem contribute to continued binge eating. As we'll see in this chapter, difficulties with relationships also seem to be relevant, and certain events and circumstances may also be influential.

Identifying Causes: A Two-Part Problem

As just stated, if binge eating problems have different outcomes in different individuals, then it is important to distinguish factors that cause the problem to start and factors that cause it to continue. For example, the factors that lead women to diet during adolescence are likely to be relevant to the development of binge eating problems, since dieting commonly precedes the onset of binge eating. In contrast, life stresses may have most impact after onset. So the question of cause actually has two parts. Turn to the question with which this chapter began, in fact, and you'll notice that it actually *is* two questions: (1) Why did this binge eating problem develop? (2) Why did it persist? So it seems natural and logical to break binge eating problems into two phases: the development phase (before onset) and the maintenance phase (after onset).

Making this distinction not only helps us understand the roles of all possible causes but also has significant practical implications for preventing and treating binge eating problems. Namely, if the goal is prevention, the task will be to identify those factors that exert their influence before onset—during the development phase—and try to stop them from operating. During treatment, in contrast, it is the factors that keep the problem going—those that are instrumental during the maintenance phase—that must be identified and dealt with, or the eating problem will tend to persist or recur.

Thus the global question "What causes binge eating problems?" should be broken down into two questions, each of which will be addressed separately in this chapter:

1. What factors increase or decrease the risk of developing a binge eating problem?
2. What factors increase or decrease the likelihood of recovery once a binge eating problem has developed?

FACTORS THAT MIGHT CAUSE BINGE EATING PROBLEMS TO BEGIN

The following factors seem to be instrumental in the onset of binge eating problems, but keep in mind that the research to date has been limited, so this information is necessarily tentative.

Social Factors

As Chapter 3 discussed, bulimia nervosa emerged in the 1970s and 1980s in those parts of the world where anorexia nervosa was already encountered: North America, northern Europe, Australia, and New Zealand. Because these are countries where it is fashionable for women to be slim and where dieting among young women is common, social factors that encourage women to diet may well contribute to its development. Key among those factors is the changing shape of fashion models. Bulimia nervosa emerged when being *extremely* thin, like the popular English model Twiggy, became fashionable.

The geographical distribution of binge eating disorder has not been studied, though it would be interesting to know whether it is the same as that for anorexia nervosa and bulimia nervosa.

Gender

Chapter 3 discussed the fact that both bulimia nervosa and binge eating disorder are much more common among women than men, though the disparity between the sexes appears to be less marked in binge eating disorder. (For more information on eating disorders in men, see the book edited by Dr. Arnold Andersen listed in Further Reading.) Why should women be at greater risk of developing binge eating problems? One major reason is likely to be the fact that dieting is so much more common among women than men; as we will discuss, dieting greatly increases the risk of developing binge eating problems.

This raises another question: Why do women tend to diet more than men? First, the social pressures to be slim are focused largely on women. Second, women are more prone than men to base their self-worth on their appearance. Both of these observations raise important wider issues concerning differences between male and female development and the competing and conflicting roles of women in Western societies. (For a feminist perspective on the cause of binge eating problems, see the article by Dr. Ruth Striegel-Moore of Wesleyan University listed in Further Reading and summarized in the box opposite.)

Ethnic Group

Again as Chapter 3 mentioned, when *patients* are considered, bulimia nervosa seems to be confined largely to Caucasian women—but clearly patient samples are subject to referral bias in terms of ethnicity. In contrast, community studies suggest that binge eating disorder occurs equally among African-American and Caucasian women. These findings need to be confirmed, however, since the studies to date have had significant shortcomings, especially in the assessment of binge eating.

Social Class

As far as *patients* are concerned, there is evidence that more people with bulimia nervosa come from middle- and upper-class backgrounds than from lower-class backgrounds. But again, this may mean only that those from middle- and upper-class backgrounds are more likely to seek treatment.

The social class distribution of binge eating disorder has yet to be defined.

Age

There is strong evidence, illustrated in Figure 13, that binge eating problems usually develop in the teenage years or early adulthood. This can probably be attributed to the fact that dieting

Femininity and Binge Eating: A Societal Perspective

In "Etiology of Binge Eating: A Developmental Perspective," Dr. Ruth H. Striegel-Moore describes how the way women define themselves and the expectations society imposes on them combine to make women in general and young women in particular vulnerable to the development of binge eating problems.

Striegel-Moore states that a woman's identity or self-definition is based on awareness of her own unique properties yet "articulated within the context of important relationships." This makes women particularly vulnerable to the opinions of others and because "physical attractiveness contributes significantly to success in the social domain, . . . it is not surprising that women make appearance and weight high priorities in their lives." This remains true even in a time when women's social roles seem to be ever expanding in range since these roles are typically represented by young, thin, highly attractive women. And unfortunate stereotypes persist: "Women who challenge traditional views of femininity, because of their political orientation (e.g., feminist) or because of their sexual orientation (e.g., lesbians) are often stereotyped as physically unattractive."

The problem with such definitions of feminine identity, the author posits, is that they lead to dieting, which may lead to binge eating. "Girls who feel insecure about their identity, especially about how they are valued by others, may focus on physical appearance because such a focus provides a concrete way to construct an identity."

Of course, as Striegel-Moore states, "for most girls, the contemporary beauty ideal is biologically unattainable." Their physical maturation takes them further from the current feminine beauty ideal. In the face of failure to achieve this ideal through dieting, girls are likely to develop low self-esteem. Thus a vicious cycle begins.

Source: Striegel-Moore RH. Etiology of binge eating: A developmental perspective. In *Binge Eating: Nature, Assessment, and Treatment.* Edited by CG Fairburn, GT Wilson. Guilford Press, New York, 1993.

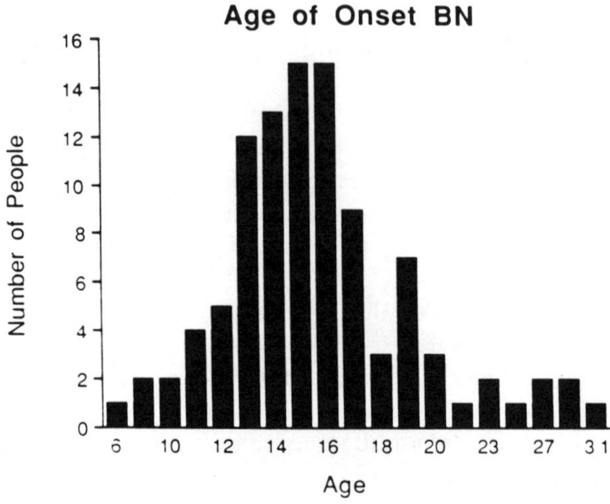

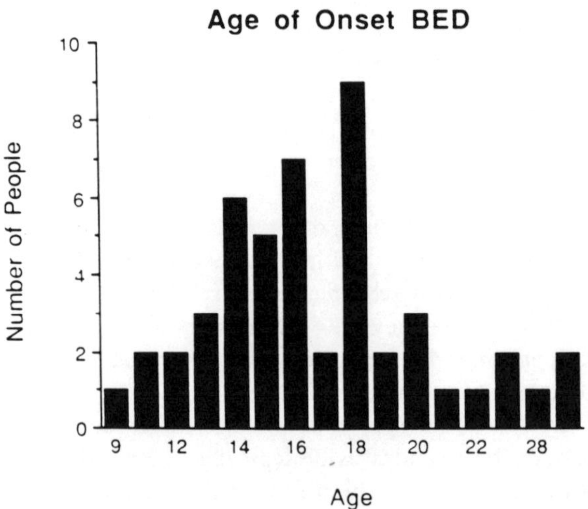

Figure 13. Age of onset of binge eating problems (BN = bulimia nervosa; BED = binge eating disorder).

among women is particularly common at this age. This, in turn, is likely to be the result of two forces. First, and as already mentioned, women are more prone than men to judge their self-worth in terms of their appearance, and this is particularly true at this age. Second, at puberty many young women develop a shape that is not considered the ideal today, as evidenced by the shape of fashion models. It's not surprising that a young woman whose developing body does not resemble the ideal might try to achieve it through dieting.

Another factor related to age is that adolescence, as we all know, presents major developmental challenges—changing appearance, fluctuations in mood, and changes in social expectations and roles. Teenagers with the personality traits that are thought to put people at risk of developing binge eating problems (see "Personality Characteristics" later in the chapter) are particularly prone to experience a sense of loss of control at this time. Some find that dieting restores their sense of control and, as a form of behavior considered socially acceptable by their peers, gives them a measurable source of achievement. For them, dieting is about self-control more than anything else, and this may remain the case for many years to come.

Certain age-dependent life changes are also relevant. A particularly important event is leaving home to go away to college. It is not at all uncommon for eating problems to develop or worsen at this time, and it is easy to see why this would happen. Not only is this a stressful transition, but for some teenagers it is the first time that they have had full control over what and when they eat. As a result some go through a phase of unchecked undereating while others overeat and gain substantial amounts of weight.

Obesity

As Chapter 5 mentioned, we now know that body shape and weight are strongly determined by genetic factors. Research findings suggest that people who develop bulimia nervosa may be at increased risk of obesity since many have been overweight in childhood and there is a raised rate of obesity among their family members. Naturally this vulnerability to obesity is likely to encourage dieting given the social pressures already mentioned. Also, having a family member with a significant weight problem may sensitize the person to "fatness," making him or her strive to avoid it by dieting. No comparable data are available on binge eating disorder although the association with obesity may be even stronger.

Eating Problems and Disorders within the Family

A number of studies have found that eating disorders run in families. This could be due to inherited factors. One way of investigating this possibility is to study twins and examine the rates of eating problems in identical and nonidentical twin pairs. Identical twins share the same genes and so should be equally at risk if the disorder is inherited, whereas nonidentical twins share, on average, half their genes like ordinary brothers and sisters. The best twin study to date (see box below) showed that there is in fact a significant genetic contribution to bulimia nervosa. Exactly what feature is inherited, however, is not known. There are many possibilities, including the tendency to be a particular weight, biological or psychological responses to dieting, and certain personality traits. No twin studies of binge eating disorder have been done to date.

The fact that eating disorders run in families does not necessarily indicate that inherited factors are wholly or even partly responsible within individual families. Aggregation within families could be due to family members "infecting" each other. A number of studies have been done of attitudes and behavior relating to food, eating, shape, and weight among the family members of those with eating disorders. To date these studies have focused on the relatives of patients with anorexia nervosa, and their findings have varied greatly. Some have found high rates of unusual behavior and attitudes; others have not.

In clinical practice accounts of apparent contagion are not uncommon. An example is mothers putting pressure on their daughters to join them on diets (see box on p. 92).

The Virginia Twin Study

In by far the largest study of its kind, interviews were conducted with 1,033 sets of female twins recruited from the Virginia Twin Registry. This is a population-based register of twins formed from a review of all birth records in the Commonwealth of Virginia. The interviews were designed to identify whether the twins had bulimia nervosa or a bulimia nervosa-like problem. The average age of the twins was 30 years.

The study found that the concordance rate in the identical twins greatly exceeded that in the nonidentical twins. In other words, if one member of an identical twin pair had bulimia nervosa, her identical sister (who shares the same genes) was much more likely to have the disorder than if the two sisters were nonidentical (i.e., no more genetically similar than ordinary sisters).

This finding provides strong evidence that genetic factors play a part in causing bulimia nervosa.

Source: Kendler KS, MacLean C, Neale M, Kessler R, Heath A, Eaves L. The genetic epidemiology of bulimia nervosa. *American Journal of Psychiatry* 1991; *148*: 1627–1637.

Psychiatric Disorders within the Family

The possibility that psychiatric disorder in the family might be a risk factor for eating disorders has also been studied. Most of this work has focused on patients with anorexia nervosa although there have been some studies of those with bulimia nervosa. The families of those with binge eating disorder have yet to be investigated.

The psychiatric disorder most widely studied so far is depression. The findings suggest that depression of clinical severity within a family increases the risk that daughters will develop an eating disorder. We do not yet know what mechanism might be responsible for this. There could be a common underlying physi-

Mothers, Daughters, and Disturbed Eating

Two groups of mothers and daughters were identified on the basis of the daughters' scores on a widely used measure of disturbed eating. There was a high-scoring group and, for comparison purposes, a low-scoring group. The average age of the daughters was 16 years and that of the mothers 43 years.

The mothers of the daughters with disturbed eating differed from the comparison mothers in the following noteworthy ways:

1. They had more disturbed eating themselves.
2. They thought that their daughters should lose more weight.
3. They were more critical of their daughters' appearance.

These findings suggest that the transmission of eating disorders within families may be, at least in part, due to contagion.

Source: Pike KM, Rodin J. Mothers, daughters, and disordered eating. *Journal of Abnormal Psychology* 1991; *100*: 198–204.

ological abnormality, such as a defect in the regulation of serotonin, a chemical thought to be involved in both depression and the control of food intake (see Chapter 5). On the other hand, it could be the influence on the child of being brought up by a depressed parent.

The other disorder to have been studied is psychoactive substance abuse (i.e., alcohol or drug abuse). As will be discussed in Chapter 7, no specific association between bulimia nervosa and substance abuse has been found. A stronger association might be predicted between binge eating disorder and substance abuse, but this has yet to be studied.

Childhood Psychiatric Disorders

As discussed in Chapter 4, people with bulimia nervosa are often clinically depressed, but this generally seems to be a consequence of the binge eating problem—it either coincides with or follows the onset of the eating problem. Recent work from my group in Oxford indicates that it is not uncommon for those with the disorder to have been depressed *prior* to its onset and that early onset of depression increases the risk of developing the disorder. No other childhood psychiatric disorders have been studied adequately in this regard.

Traumatic Events and Experiences during Childhood

Clinicians who work with those with binge eating problems cannot fail to notice how common it is for traumatic events to have occurred during their patients' childhoods. Deaths, separations, parental disharmony, physical illnesses, teasing, and bullying all seem to occur with disturbing frequency. However, it is not yet clear whether such events occur any more often among these patients than among those with other psychiatric disorders.

Sexual abuse is the one event to have been studied in some detail. Initially it was thought that the rate of childhood sexual abuse was especially high among those with bulimia nervosa. However, research from Leicester University in England suggested that the rate of childhood sexual abuse among patients with eating disorders is no higher than that among patients with other psychiatric disorders (see box on p. 94). A study from my group in Oxford compared the rates of sexual abuse among three groups recruited direct from the community: women with no psychiatric disorder, women with a psychiatric disorder other than an eating disorder, and women with bulimia nervosa. Since the three groups were recruited from the community, the possible biasing effect of studying only those who seek treatment was avoided. The findings indicated that there is an association between childhood sexual abuse and the subsequent development of an eating disorder, but probably not a specific one; those with other psychiatric disorders were just as likely to have been sexually abused in the past. Thus the evidence suggests that women who have been sexually abused in childhood are at increased risk of psychiatric disturbance in general and not eating disorders in particular. While this finding indicates that the specific role of sexual abuse is limited, it does not of course diminish the importance of sexual abuse as an etiological factor in individual cases.

Personality Characteristics

As first mentioned in Chapter 4, people with certain personality characteristics seem particularly prone to develop binge eating problems. Most of the research on this topic has focused on pa-

Sexual Abuse and Eating Disorders

In the first study of its kind, researchers from Leicester University in England compared the rates of childhood sexual abuse among female patients with eating disorders and female patients with other psychiatric disorders.

The study had two stages. First the women completed a self-report questionnaire concerning their childhood experience of events that could be construed as sexual abuse. Then each was interviewed by a female investigator to clarify the nature of the events reported.

Overall it was found that 31% of the women with eating disorders had experienced such an event, compared with 50% of the women with other psychiatric disorders. Subdividing the events in terms of their nature, the perpetrator, and the age at which they occurred did not alter the overall pattern of findings.

These results suggest that the rate of childhood sexual abuse is no higher among those with eating disorders than among those with other psychiatric disorders. This finding has since been confirmed by other research groups.

Source: Palmer RL, Oppenheimer R. Childhood experiences with adults: A comparison of women with eating disorders and those with other diagnoses. *International Journal of Eating Disorders* 1992; *12*: 359–364.

tients with anorexia nervosa and is thus more relevant to bulimia nervosa than binge eating disorder.

Apparently those who develop anorexia nervosa are unusually compliant and conscientious as children. They are often somewhat shy and solitary, and they may have difficulty mixing with other children. In addition, they tend to be competitive and achievement oriented. They set themselves high standards and drive themselves to meet them. These specific traits seem to be the precursors of the low self-esteem and perfectionism seen in many patients with anorexia nervosa and bulimia nervosa.

Exploratory psychotherapy often confirms these findings. Dr. Michael Strober from UCLA, a leading expert on personality and eating disorders, has stated that a detailed investigation of these patients' inner world reveals "the omnipresent fear of seeming weak, inadequate and average; the inability to take pleasure in leisure; a reluctance to confront risks and novelty, to engage in uninhibited spontaneous action, or to assert feelings; and the experiencing of impulses and desires as wasteful distractions to achieving higher moral objectives." Dr. Strober argues that personality characteristics of this type result in these people being "hopelessly ill prepared" for the developmental demands of adolescence.

The personality characteristics of those with binge eating disorder have not been studied to date, but work with patients implies that some of the same traits are involved. In particular, people with binge eating disorder seem to have problems with assertiveness and low self-esteem.

As mentioned earlier, there is a subgroup among those with binge eating problems that has difficulties in general with impulse control, and often these difficulties were evident in childhood.

Dieting

Chapter 4 introduced the connection between binge eating and dieting and showed that both are part of a cycle that tends to perpetuate itself. However, dieting also increases the risk of developing a binge eating problem; indeed it is the most well substantiated risk factor. For example, one study (see box below) showed that among teenagers dieters were eight times as likely to develop bulimia nervosa as nondieters. Still, we know that the majority of those who diet do not develop eating problems. Therefore other factors of the type already mentioned must combine with dieting to increase the risk of developing binge eating problems. Also, it may be that only certain forms of dieting are prone to put people at risk.

The Bottom Line: No Single Cause

There is no single cause of binge eating problems. It does seem that in many cases dieting plays an important direct role in causing binge eating (see Chapter 4). The close relationship between dieting and binge eating seems to account for the geographical distribution of bulimia nervosa, the fact that women are most at risk for binge eating problems, and the age of onset of these problems. On the other hand, we know that binge eating is not *invariably* preceded by dieting; nor do all dieters develop binge eating problems. This means that other factors—social, psychological, or

Dieting as a Risk Factor

One hundred and seventy-six girls from 8 state schools in London were interviewed on two occasions 12 months apart. At the outset their average age was 15 years, and a third (35%) were judged to be dieters.

When reassessed 12 months later, a significant number of the dieters were found to have developed bulimia nervosa. The investigators calculated that dieters were 8 times more likely than nondieters to develop the disorder.

Source: Patton GC, Johnson-Sabine E, Wood K, Mann AH, Wakeling A. Abnormal eating attitudes in London schoolgirls—A prospective epidemiological study: Outcome at twelve month follow-up. *Psychological Medicine* 1990; *20*: 383–394.

physical, on their own or in combination with dieting—have a major influence.

FACTORS THAT MIGHT KEEP BINGE EATING PROBLEMS ACTIVE

Little research has been done on how binge eating problems change over time and what factors influence their course. So it's difficult to say what causes these problems to persist, what makes them cease, and what leads to a recurrence. Several factors do appear to be important, however.

Ongoing Dieting

In Chapter 4 I described various ways in which dieting makes people prone to binge. If the dieting is "extreme" (that is, the dieter exercises such restraint that he or she eats little), strong physiological pressures to eat will come to bear. And if the dieting is "strict" (the dieter sets highly specific dietary goals and holds a perfectionist attitude toward them), he or she will tend to swing between dieting and binge eating with each promoting the other. Through these mechanisms, ongoing dieting seems to maintain binge eating problems. It is for this reason that many treatments focus on eliminating or moderating dieting (see Chapter 8 and Part II). Interestingly, dieting seems to encourage episodes of overeating even in people who do not binge. A large body of laboratory research has identified among dieters a so-called counter-regulation effect—the tendency of dieters to abandon their diet and overeat under a variety of circumstances.

Various factors encourage dieting, the main ones being the drive to exert self-control mentioned earlier and the influence of concerns about appearance and weight. These concerns are reinforced by Western society's current preference for a thin body shape. People who have been overweight in the past may be particularly likely to diet for fear of regaining the lost weight, and their efforts may be encouraged by friends and relatives.

Vomiting and Misusing Laxatives

Both of these methods of weight control tend to encourage binge eating since belief in their effectiveness neutralizes a major deterrent to binge eating, namely the fear of weight gain. In bulimia nervosa, where such methods are common, a number of interacting vicious circles therefore promote continued binge eating (see Figure 14). These were discussed in Chapter 4.

Relationships, Events, and Circumstances

A variety of events and circumstances may influence the course of binge eating problems. Personal relationships are particularly important in this regard. For example, establishing a close and accepting relationship with a partner may improve self-esteem, decrease concerns about shape and weight, and remove some sources of stress, thereby promoting recovery. The breakdown of a relationship can have the reverse effect. While no findings are yet available, research being conducted at Oxford may yield more information on this subject in the future.

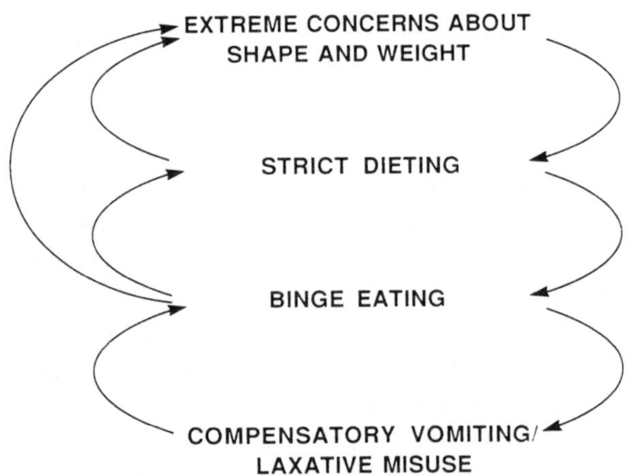

Figure 14. Vicious circles that maintain binge eating.

Pregnancy

As Chapter 4 discussed, pregnancy has a particularly revealing effect on binge eating problems. Some pregnant women no longer feel accountable for their weight and therefore feel no need to diet; indeed fear of harming the fetus puts pressure on them not to diet. This lessening of any tendency to diet may account for the finding that binge eating problems tend to improve during pregnancy, sometimes going away altogether. Unfortunately, many of these women resume dieting shortly after childbirth, and this may explain in part why relapse is so common.

THE DESIRE TO CHANGE

As mentioned, regrettably little research has been done on the factors that influence the course of binge eating problems. Yet such research is needed, not simply to further our understanding of these problems but also to assist in the development of new approaches to treatment (see Chapter 8).

The factors just discussed do not constitute an exhaustive list. In fact our discussion of the factors contributing to the persistence of binge eating problems omitted one key factor, namely the motivation to change. Some people seem to have little desire to change. They accept their binge eating problem and adjust their life around it. In such cases the problem tends to persist. Others make a decision to change, to make a fresh start. Interestingly, having made such a decision, some are able to change on their own. Others, however, cannot. They need outside help.

What stimulates people to decide to make a fresh start has not been studied, but it should be. One of my hopes, as author of this book, is that it might provide readers with binge eating problems with just such a stimulus.

CHAPTER 7

Binge Eating and Addiction

WHEN CHAPTER 6 CONSIDERED the causes of binge eating, one question was not addressed: Is binge eating an addiction? If you've ever experienced the loss of control associated with bingeing, that question may very well have crossed your mind. Or, especially if you live in the United States, where the issue has received the most attention, you may have read about it. With terms such as *compulsive overeating* and *food addict* permeating so much of the public discussion of binge eating, it is hardly surprising that the characterization of binge eating as a form of addiction has become popular. In fact this theory has gained such a strong following that it is the basis for certain prominent treatment programs.

For that reason, it is important to understand how addiction might be involved in binge eating. If it is not an influence in binge eating problems, then treatment schemes based on that premise may well not succeed. This chapter therefore focuses on three main questions:

1. Is it appropriate to view binge eating as an addiction?
2. Is there any relationship between true addictions such as alcohol and drug abuse and binge eating?

3. What does our knowledge of this relationship tell us about how binge eating problems should be treated?

THE THEORY OF BINGE EATING AS AN ADDICTION

> OA believes that compulsive overeating is a threefold disease: physical, emotional and spiritual. We regard it as an addiction which, like alcoholism and drug abuse, can be arrested but not cured.
>
> —Overeaters Anonymous leaflet

According to the theory that binge eating is a form of addiction—called the addiction "model" of binge eating—binge eating is the result of an underlying illness or disease akin to that responsible for alcoholism. People who binge are biologically vulnerable to certain foods (typically sugar and starches) and as a result become "addicted" to them. These foods are regarded as "toxic." Vulnerable individuals are unable to control their intake of these foods, so their consumption rises progressively. Since the vulnerability is biologically based, they can never be cured of the problem (or "illness"): Rather, they have to learn to accept it and adjust their lives accordingly.

Is the addiction model valid? As Dr. G. Terence Wilson points out, "The concept of addiction has been debased by promiscuous and imprecise usage to describe virtually any form of repetitive behavior." Some of us, we are told, are "love addicts"; others are "TV addicts." The result is that it is no longer clear at all what it means to be addicted. When the word is used in this loose, all-embracing way, most of us could be said to be "addicted" to something or other. Obviously, then, we must be particularly cautious in defining binge eating or any other behavior as an addiction.

Still, there are some similarities between binge eating and the classic addictions involving alcohol and drug abuse, and many people rely on these similarities to support the addiction model of binge eating. They point out that whether the behavior is alcohol/drug abuse or binge eating, the person

- Has cravings or urges to engage in the behavior
- Feels a loss of control over the behavior
- Is preoccupied with thoughts about the behavior
- Might use the behavior to relieve tension and negative feelings
- Denies the severity of the problem
- Attempts to keep the problem secret
- Persists in the behavior despite its adverse effects
- Often makes repeated unsuccessful attempts to stop

These similarities are, however, superficial. They are interesting, and some are relevant to treatment—for example, the use of the behavior to deal with tension—but the fact that things are similar or have properties in common does not make them the same. And focusing exclusively on these similarities, as is often done, distracts from the differences between these behaviors, differences that are both central to the understanding of them and central to their successful treatment.

The differences between binge eating and substance abuse are most obvious in the case of bulimia nervosa:

- *The inherent drive to avoid the behavior.* People with bulimia nervosa are continually trying to restrict their food intake (see Chapter 4). What distresses them about their binge eating is that it represents their failure to control their eating and carries the risk of weight gain. There is no equivalent phenomenon in alcohol (or drug) abuse. Those who abuse alcohol have no inherent drive to avoid alcohol, against which the excessive drinking takes place. In fact a major goal of addiction treatment programs is to instill in the addict the determination not to engage in the addictive behavior. In bulimia nervosa, in contrast, that determination already exists in the form of the strong desire to control food intake. Indeed, the drive to control eating is a problem in its own right that has to be tackled in treatment (see Chapter 8 and Part II).

- *Fear of engaging in the behavior.* In bulimia nervosa, accompanying the drive to diet is a set of attitudes toward shape and weight characterized by an intense fear of weight gain and fatness and, in some, a pursuit of thinness. Issues regarding appearance and weight dominate these peoples' lives (see Chapter 4). They judge their self-worth almost exclusively in terms of their appearance and weight, and these attitudes play an important role in perpetuating the disorder (see Chapter 6). There is no equivalent phenomenon in alcohol abuse. Those who drink excessively show no fear of getting drunk and no pursuit of sobriety.

In other words, the desire to *restrict* eating encourages those with bulimia nervosa to binge, whereas those addicted to alcohol or drugs are not vulnerable to abuse of these substances *because* they wish to avoid them. The differing mechanisms involved in binge eating and substance abuse thus point to two diametrically opposed approaches to their treatment: In binge eating treatment should focus on *moderating* self-restraint; treatment for addiction should focus on *strengthening* it.

On the other hand, binge eating does occur among individuals who do not diet particularly intensely, specifically those with binge eating disorder. The binge eating of these people, many of whom are overweight, is not driven by dieting, or at least not to the same extent. Difficulties coping with stress seem to be more important. So perhaps more of an overlap exists between the mechanisms driving their binge eating and those driving alcohol or drug abuse.

THE RELATIONSHIP BETWEEN BINGE EATING AND SUBSTANCE ABUSE

Even if binge eating is not itself an addiction, are the similarities between binge eating and substance abuse indicative of an association between the two? Could both problems be caused by a single underlying abnormality? To answer these questions, studies have been done to determine how often and under what circumstances the two problems appear in the same person.

Substance Abuse among People with Binge Eating Problems

While proponents of the addiction model of binge eating often state that the rates of alcohol and drug abuse are disproportionately high among those with binge eating problems, the research findings in fact have been inconsistent. For example, while doctors at the University of Minnesota have reported that over a third of their patients with bulimia nervosa have a history of problems with alcohol or other drugs, among Oxford patients the figure is more like 10 percent. Before we can decide whether either of these figures (or anything in between) is actually a high rate of substance abuse, we need to figure out why such discrepancies exist in the first place:

1. The inconsistent findings could be the result of differences in local treatment services. The Minnesota research group, for example, has a reputation for studying substance abuse. So it might attract a disproportionate number of those with both problems, thereby obtaining an inflated figure for how often they occur together.
2. The discrepancy could be a function of the relative rates of alcohol and drug problems in the local general population. That is, if over a third of the general population in Minnesota abuses alcohol or drugs, as opposed to only 10 percent of the general population in Oxford, the discrepancy may be caused simply by where the two groups of patients live.

Without such facts in hand, we cannot determine whether there is any true discrepancy between the two figures. Let's say, though, that the available facts suggested that the real rate of alcohol and drug abuse among patients with bulimia nervosa was in between the rates revealed by the two studies: 20 percent. To decide whether 20 percent can be considered "high," we still must consider several factors:

1. The figures obtained by researchers are based on *patients* with bulimia nervosa (that is, those who have sought treatment). It would not be surprising if patients had artificially high rates of alcohol and drug abuse when compared to individuals who have not sought help, because people who have two problems are more likely to seek help than those with only one.
2. To determine whether there is a *specific* association between alcohol and drug abuse and binge eating problems, we have to know the rates of alcohol and drug abuse among those with other psychological problems, such as anxiety or depression. If the rate of alcohol or drug abuse is raised among those with binge eating problems, but is equally high among those with anxiety or depression, the association cannot be considered specific. In other words, those who have psychological problems of any sort are prone to abuse alcohol or drugs.
3. Again, whether the rate of alcohol or drug abuse is relatively high among patients with bulimia nervosa depends on how the rate among these people compares to the rate among the general population. A rate of 20 percent among patients with bulimia nervosa would have vastly different implications when compared to general-population rates of 5 percent, 20 percent, and 50 percent.

There is only one way to resolve the matter. It is to study the rates of coexistence of these problems using community rather than patient samples. My colleagues at Oxford and I are engaged in a study of this type, but its findings are not yet available.

As matters stand, there are insufficient grounds for concluding that alcohol and drug abuse is especially common among those who binge eat, and there are certainly no grounds for claiming that there is a specific association between them.

Binge Eating Problems among Those with Substance Abuse Problems

If there is in fact a specific association between binge eating and substance abuse, those with alcohol and drug addiction should have a raised rate of binge eating problems. Only recently have researchers begun to investigate this issue, and the results of their studies do suggest an increased rate of eating problems and of binge eating in particular. To date, however, only those seeking treatment have been studied (the largest such study is described in the box below), and again, patient samples may be atypical. In addition, there is evidence that the rate of eating problems among patients with other psychological problems is also high, raising the possibility that the association is a nonspecific one. So it is important to exercise caution in drawing conclusions; evidence for a specific association is still lacking.

Family Studies

Several studies have reported a higher-than-expected rate of substance abuse among the relatives of patients with bulimia nervosa. This finding is interesting but, like the others already mentioned, difficult to interpret. The rates seem no higher than those among the relatives of patients with other psychiatric disorders. The rates of eating problems among the relatives of those with substance abuse have not been studied. Again, all the work has focused on patient rather than community samples.

The Relationship between the Disorders over Time

To understand the relationship between two disorders, it is important to know whether one tends to lead to the other or vice versa. Studies of alcoholic patients who have an eating problem suggest that the latter develops first. This finding is difficult to evaluate, however, since eating problems typically begin at an earlier age than alcohol problems. Interestingly, patients who have both an alcohol and an eating problem also tend to be

Eating Disorders and Alcohol Abuse: Findings from Japan

The subjects in this study were 3,592 patients (336 females and 3,256 males) admitted to the National Institute on Alcoholism, Kurihama National Hospital, Japan, between 1982 and 1988. On admission each was screened for an eating disorder, and possible cases were subsequently interviewed in detail following their recovery from alcohol withdrawal symptoms.

The main findings were as follows:

1. Eleven percent of the female patients had an eating disorder. Eating disorders were most common among the young patients with 72% of those under the age of 30 years being affected.
2. Eating disorders were uncommon among the men (0.2% were affected).
3. Bulimia nervosa was the most common eating disorder detected.
4. In only 10% of the cases in which the two disorders coexisted did the alcohol problem develop before the eating disorder. In the females with an eating disorder, the average age of onset of the eating disorder was 19.7 years, whereas the problem drinking started on average at 24.6 years. A similar pattern was observed among the men.
5. There was no evidence that eating disorders and alcohol problems alternated within individuals over time.

This study is by far the largest of the studies on this topic. The findings are in line with those of the other studies, although the rate of eating problems reported by this study is higher.

Source: Higuchi S, Suzuki K, Yamada K, Parrish K, Kono H. Alcoholics with eating disorders: Prevalence and clinical course. *British Journal of Psychiatry* 1993; *162*: 403–406.

younger than those who have an alcohol problem alone. This suggests that eating problems might somehow bring forward alcohol problems.

The Effects of Treatment

If one abnormality underlies both binge eating and substance abuse, then the successful treatment of one of these problems might lead to the emergence of the other (unless the underlying abnormality had also been corrected). This phenomenon is sometimes called *symptom substitution*. There is no evidence that it occurs. While we know nothing about the development of eating problems among those who have been treated successfully for substance abuse, we do have information on the outcome of those who have received treatment for bulimia nervosa. Substance abuse is uncommon.

The Myth of the Addiction Model

Based on what we know, it is clear that an association between binge eating and psychoactive substance abuse exists among certain individuals. *Whether the disorders themselves are linked, however, is not known,* and we certainly have no evidence that any such association is *specific.*

Clearly, then, the addiction model of binge eating—which assumes a specific association—is not supported by the facts. Only superficial similarities exist between binge eating and substance abuse. Nor is there evidence that binge eating is the product of an underlying biological abnormality. The idea that people can become "addicted" to certain foods (at least in the technical sense of the word) is far-fetched.

IMPLICATIONS FOR TREATMENT

> Our goal is to abstain from compulsive overeating one day at a time. We do this through daily personal contact, meetings and by following the twelve-step program of Alcoholics Anonymous,

changing only the words "alcohol" and "alcoholic" to "food" and "compulsive overeater."

—Overeaters Anonymous leaflet

Current understanding of the relationship between binge eating and substance abuse is so limited that it has little relevance to treatment. One point is clear, however: There are no grounds for claiming that binge eating is an addiction. Given that, is it appropriate to treat it as one? In fact the principles underlying addiction-oriented treatment are at odds with the approach that has proved to be most effective (see Chapter 8).

Treatment, according to the addiction model, should be based on the approach used by Alcoholics Anonymous and other related groups for helping those with alcohol problems. This is the so-called twelve-step approach. Four features distinguish this approach from the most successful form of treatment, a psychological treatment called *cognitive-behavioral therapy,* which is described in Chapter 8 and Part II:

1. *Twelve-step approach: The disorder is an illness for which there is no cure.* A book of daily readings for members of Overeaters Anonymous says, "It is the experience of recovering compulsive overeaters that the illness is progressive. The disease does not get better; it gets worse. Even while we abstain, the illness progresses."

   Cognitive-behavioral approach: Recovery is well within the reach of most people. Long-term follow-up studies of bulimia nervosa indicate that full recovery is common and that with appropriate treatment the great majority of people improve substantially (see Chapter 8).

2. *Twelve-step approach: Immediate abstinence is paramount.* The focus is on stopping binge eating as rapidly as possible, and group pressure may be applied to serve this end. In some meetings, abstinent participants are identified and praised, whereas those who have not been abstinent are given little or no opportunity to speak: Indeed, they may be asked to leave.

Cognitive-behavioral approach: Emphasis on the immediate cessation of bingeing is neither reasonable nor realistic. The abstinence approach is heartless and unreasonable. While with good advice and support many people can rapidly stop binge eating, many others cannot. It may take them weeks or months to get to this point. There is no evidence that rapid cessation of binge eating is associated with a better long-term outcome than more gradual change. Indeed, more gradual change may be preferable since it provides opportunities to develop skills for dealing with situations that might otherwise lead to relapse. The cognitive-behavioral approach places no emphasis on the immediate cessation of binge eating.

3. *Twelve-step approach: A major strategy for achieving abstinence is an additional form of abstinence, the total lifelong avoidance of the ("toxic") foods that trigger episodes of binge eating.*

   Cognitive-behavioral approach: Food avoidance should be eliminated, not encouraged. As discussed earlier, the view that certain foods are toxic and somehow cause people to binge has no basis in fact. Clinical and experimental evidence indicates that it is the very attempts to avoid these foods that makes people vulnerable to bingeing (see Chapter 4). It is for this reason that the cognitive-behavioral approach focuses on eliminating food avoidance rather than encouraging it. Professor Walter Vandereycken from Leuven in Belgium has called the emphasis of twelve-step programs on avoiding foods "anorexic skills training"; if successful, it might convert people who binge into anorexics, an outcome they might find attractive in principle but a nightmare in reality.

4. *Twelve-step approach: One is either in control or out of control, foods are safe or toxic, one is abstinent or not.* Underpinning the abstinence approach is an all-or-nothing mentality (see Chapter 4).

   Cognitive-behavioral approach: Black-and-white thinking is a problem that must be tackled. To take one example, an all-

> or-nothing view of progress after treatment encourages people to regard any setback as a "relapse" rather than a "lapse." Dr. G. Alan Marlatt from the University of Washington in Seattle has shown, with respect to alcohol abuse, that this way of thinking leads people to give up when there is no need for them to do so. All-or-nothing thinking is common among people who binge, and it seems to contribute to their problems (see Chapter 4). So, rather than reinforcing this way of thinking, as in the abstinence approach, it is important to help people recognize and moderate it (see Part II).

There is, of course, more to addiction-based treatments than I have presented. Their greatest strength is the high level of support and fellowship that they provide. That, combined with the simplicity of their message, makes them of great value to some people. However, the "bottom line" must be effectiveness. The twelve-step approach to binge eating problems has yet to be evaluated properly, whereas a great deal is known about the effectiveness of other forms of treatment. These are the subject of the next chapter.

CHAPTER 8

Treatment of Binge Eating Problems

YOU HAVE NOW LEARNED what we know so far about binge eating problems—how we define them, what types of psychological, social, and physical factors are involved in causing them, and who, as far as the research has been able to discern, is affected. You should also be aware by now that what we don't know is substantial, perhaps especially in the area of cause. Why someone you know began binge eating and why that person continues to do so may still be a mystery to you. Now, however, you can probably appreciate that the complex combination of factors that can result in binge eating problems may also prevent or at least delay many people from getting help.

The fact that people with binge eating problems commonly postpone seeking help is all the more regrettable given that effective forms of treatment are available. We have learned a lot about the treatment of these problems over the last twenty years. While much of this research has focused on bulimia nervosa, it now seems that treatments that have shown promise in this context also benefit those with binge eating disorder.

This chapter outlines our current knowledge about the treatment of binge eating problems. All forms of treatment are discussed, but particular emphasis is placed on the use of antidepressant drugs and a specific form of short-term psychotherapy called *cognitive-behavioral therapy* since both of these approaches have been the focus of particularly intense research efforts.

The ability of treatment to produce enduring change is paramount because binge eating problems tend to be well established before people seek help. Many people pursue treatment after having experienced five or more years of unremitting problems, and if they have received any treatment in the past, the benefits have often been short-lived. For this reason the true test of any treatment for binge eating is whether it results in lasting improvement. Changes that endure for only weeks or months are of limited significance.

One preliminary question that may occur to those whose eating problems have persisted despite attempts at treatment is whether hospitalization will be necessary. In fact, hospitalization is rarely necessary. Both clinical and research experience indicate that the great majority of people with binge eating problems may be treated as outpatients.

In fact, hospitalization not only may be unnecessary but also may be counterproductive. People tend to stop binge eating soon after entering the hospital, and a naive therapist might conclude mistakenly that hospitalization is helping the person overcome the problem. In fact, however, people tend to stop bingeing when in the hospital because it is a foreign environment where access to food is limited, because they are protected from many of the stresses of everyday life that tend to trigger binges, and because privacy is often restricted. So in reality their binge eating is merely in abeyance and is likely to return upon leaving the hospital.

The best inpatient programs try to prevent relapses after discharge by helping people develop skills for dealing with the factors that lead them to binge. The trouble is that the hospital is not a good environment in which to do this. The therapist and patient need to tackle the binge eating problem as it normally exists, and that means in the outside world.

Of course, there are certain circumstances under which admission to a hospital is advisable. Five stand out:

1. Some people with binge eating problems are so depressed that they cannot make use of outpatient treatment.
2. Some are suicidal and so need the protection of a hospital.
3. In some cases the person's physical health is a cause for concern (see Chapter 5).
4. It is probably wise for those in the early stages of pregnancy to come into the hospital if their eating habits are severely disturbed, because there is some evidence that the miscarriage rate may be raised (see Chapter 5).
5. Hospitalization is also indicated for those whose eating problem has not responded to appropriate outpatient treatment.

In practice, these circumstances apply to probably less than 5 percent of cases. There is, however, one other reason for considering hospitalization that could be pertinent to a large number of people. Namely, in countries without socialized medicine, insurance coverage may provide the only available financial means for paying for treatment, and many insurance policies cover mainly inpatient care. Under these circumstances, individuals may have little choice but to enter a hospital.

Whatever the reason for hospitalization, it should always be viewed as preparation for outpatient treatment so that the changes achieved in the hospital can be transferred successfully to the patient's own environment.

ANTIDEPRESSANT DRUGS

Interest in using antidepressant drugs to treat binge eating problems began in 1982 with the publication of two scientific papers describing a favorable response in patients with bulimia nervosa. The following year the findings of two treatment trials were published. In these trials the effects of an antidepressant drug were compared with those of a placebo. One of these studies found the antidepressant drug markedly superior to the placebo; the other did not. Nevertheless, enthusiasm grew, fueled by the 1984 publication of a book titled *New Hope for Binge Eaters,* in which Drs. Harrison Pope and James Hudson from Harvard, the researchers who conducted the study with the positive findings, argued strongly for the use of these drugs.

Since the publication of this book much more research has been conducted, and the facts have become clearer. All major types of antidepressant drugs have been studied, and there have been three positive findings:

1. Within a few weeks of treatment there is, on average, a 50 to 60 percent reduction in the frequency of binge eating.
2. Associated with this reduction are an equivalent fall in the frequency of vomiting, an improvement in mood and sense of control over eating, and decreased preoccupation with eating.
3. The antidepressant drug effect is just as likely to occur whether or not the patient is depressed to start with.

Unfortunately, problems have also emerged. The first is that some antidepressants, particularly drugs like phenelzine (Nardil), have troublesome side effects. Most of the unwanted effects are not medically serious, but the use of one drug, bupropion (Wellbutrin), was associated with epileptic fits in some patients. The second problem is that many people are reluctant to take the drugs because they do not see them as an appropriate treatment for their problem. This attitude, which has been confirmed by my own clinical experience and that of many others, explains why researchers have found it easier to recruit people for studies of psychological treatments than for drug studies. But it is the third problem that is most significant. This is that there are serious doubts about whether the beneficial effects last. As already mentioned, short-lived treatment effects are of limited value when helping people with binge eating problems, yet most of the antidepressant drug studies have been short-term—often only eight weeks long. Recent findings, including those of a longer-term study described in the box on page 116, indicate that many people who have benefited from these drugs subsequently start binge eating again, whether or not they continue taking the drug.

The research has also shown that antidepressant drugs have a selective effect on binge eating problems. While many of those

Antidepressant Drugs and Bulimia Nervosa: Do the Beneficial Effects Last?

Almost all the studies of the use of antidepressant drugs in the treatment of binge eating problems have been short in duration, most lasting just 8 weeks. This is a short time given that binge eating problems tend to be long lasting.

A research group lead by Dr B. Timothy Walsh of Columbia University has studied the longer-term effects of these drugs. Patients with bulimia nervosa were first treated for 6 weeks with the antidepressant drug desipramine. Those who responded continued on the drug for 16 weeks longer. At that point those who had not relapsed either stayed on the drug or were switched over to inert placebo pills (without their knowledge but with their prior consent).

The results were disappointing. Although the patients who received 6 weeks of desipramine experienced, on average, a 47% reduction in their frequency of binge eating, they were continuing to binge on average 4.3 times weekly. Only 41% were judged to have responded sufficiently well to justify continuing the drug. Of these, almost a third (29%) relapsed over the following 4 months, a figure equivalent to that obtained by an earlier but smaller study.

This study shows that antidepressant drugs have a limited beneficial effect. While the frequency of binge eating falls in the short term, most people continue to binge at an appreciable rate. And if a longer-term perspective is taken, the results are modest indeed.

Source: Walsh BT, Hadigan BA, Devlin MJ, Gladis M, Roose SP. Long-term outcome of antidepressant treatment for bulimia nervosa. *American Journal of Psychiatry* 1991; *148*: 1206–1212.

who take the drugs start to binge (and also vomit or misuse laxatives) less frequently, they tend to diet just as intensely. For example, a study from Stanford University of patients with bulimia nervosa found that the average daily food intake outside binges was just 1,017 calories before treatment and only 1,033 calories after treatment—about half the normal daily calorie intake for women. Perhaps, then, it's the persistence of such dieting that explains why the benefits of antidepressants often do not last.

Awareness that antidepressant drugs are of limited value in the longer term has led to waning enthusiasm for their use. Even those research groups whose primary interest was in evaluating the effectiveness of these drugs are now turning to evaluating psychological treatments instead. Simultaneously, the organizers of international conferences on eating disorders are reporting that they are receiving fewer and fewer papers on their use. Antidepressant drugs are not the "new hope for binge eaters" as originally suggested.

What about other drugs? The effects of drugs such as lithium, drugs used for epilepsy such as phenytoin and carbamazepine, and appetite suppressants such as fenfluramine have all been studied, but none looks promising. Therefore, none of these are recommended.

COGNITIVE-BEHAVIORAL THERAPY

The experience of clinicians and researchers strongly suggests that the real hope for those with binge eating problems lies in psychological treatment. The most effective approach to date is a specific form of short-term psychotherapy designed originally for patients with bulimia nervosa and recently adapted for those with binge eating disorder. Developed by the author in the late 1970s, this treatment borrowed techniques from the then relatively new cognitive therapy for depression and from behavioral approaches to the treatment of obesity. After trial and error over several years, it took its present form by 1981.

This approach to treating binge eating problems has received great interest for several reasons:

1. It helps the great majority of people with binge eating problems. It has been studied at most major research centers—in the United States, Canada, the United Kingdom, Germany, Australia, and New Zealand—with equivalent positive results. No other treatment has proved as successful.
2. It is readily accepted by most patients, who see it as relevant and appropriate.
3. A clinician's treatment "manual" has been available for some time, making it easy for therapists to adopt the approach.
4. It is neither unusually long nor difficult to reproduce, making it easy to research. Typically it is conducted on a one-to-one outpatient basis and involves roughly twenty therapy sessions over four to five months.

A form of what is currently called *cognitive-behavioral therapy,* this approach is ideally suited to the treatment of binge eating problems because its cognitive elements address the cognitive aspects of these problems—the extreme concern about shape and weight, perfectionism and all-or-nothing thinking, and low self-esteem—while its behavioral components tackle the disturbed eating habits. The fact that the cognitive techniques were originally developed to treat depression implies no connection between binge eating problems and depression; the reason these techniques were adapted for use in treating eating problems was that they appeared capable of producing cognitive change. (In contrast, those who originally advocated the use of antidepressant drugs justified their use by arguing that there was in fact a link between bulimia nervosa and depression—some even said bulimia nervosa was a form of depression—a view since shown to be largely fallacious.) While the cognitive-behavioral approach to treating binge eating problems is similar, in principle, to cognitive therapy for depression, the focus and procedures are very different.

The core elements of the treatment are listed in Table 7. The treatment is designed to erode the problem progressively, using a carefully planned *sequence of interventions*. It begins with the use of behavioral and educational techniques to help the person regain control over eating, a key element being helping the person establish a pattern of regular eating through the day. This tends to displace many binges. However, the increase in control that results is brittle since most people remain highly vulnerable to bingeing. Therefore, in the second stage of treatment the emphasis switches to reducing this vulnerability by tackling the tendency to diet and those problematic ways of thinking that maintain binge eating (discussed in Chapters 4 and

Table 7. The Core Elements of the Cognitive-Behavioral Approach

Stage One

Recording in detail all eating at the time that it occurs, together with relevant thoughts and feelings
Introducing a pattern of regular eating, thereby displacing many binges
Using alternative behavior to help resist urges to binge
Receiving education about food, eating, shape, and weight

Stage Two

Introducing avoided foods into the diet and gradually eliminating other forms of strict dieting
Developing skills for dealing with difficulties that might otherwise trigger binges
Identifying and changing problematic ways of thinking
Considering the origins of the binge eating problem and the role of family and social factors

Stage Three

Planning for the future, including having realistic expectations and strategies to use should problems recur

Source: Fairburn CG, Marcus MD, Wilson GT. Cognitive-behavioral therapy for binge eating and bulimia nervosa: A comprehensive treatment manual. In *Binge Eating: Nature, Assessment, and Treatment.* Edited by CG Fairburn, GT Wilson. Guilford Press, New York, 1993.

6). The final stage involves a review of what procedures were most helpful so the person can draw up a plan for tackling any future difficulties.

The cognitive-behavioral approach to treating binge eating problems has been studied extensively over the last fifteen years. Major research projects conducted at Rutgers, Stanford, Minnesota, Vermont, Toronto, Edinburgh, Cambridge, and Oxford have produced remarkably consistent findings. Like antidepressant drugs, these studies have found that cognitive-behavioral therapy has an immediate effect on the frequency of binge eating. Even more encouraging, though, is that the effect is not only greater in magnitude than with antidepressant drugs but also longer-lasting. For example, the most recent study from my group in Oxford obtained a 90 percent average reduction by the end of treatment that was maintained one and six years later.

The studies have also shown that the decrease in frequency of binge eating is accompanied by improvements in mood, concentration, and sense of control over eating, as with antidepressant drugs. But in addition, concerns about shape and weight lessen in intensity, as does the dieting. Perhaps this is why, in contrast to treatment with antidepressant drugs, the changes achieved with cognitive-behavioral therapy seem to endure.

The potential of cognitive-behavioral therapy for treating binge eating disorder, on the other hand, is not as certain. Researchers at Stanford have had some success in a group setting, but there was a tendency to relapse. Researchers from Pittsburgh are also getting promising results using a modified version of the treatment on a one-to-one basis, and in this case relapse appears not to be such a problem. Both groups have focused on people who are also overweight, yet neither has found that treatment has a significant effect on weight. This may be because the effects on weight take a long time to emerge or because treatment is not succeeding in tackling these people's general tendency to overeat, mentioned in Chapter 4. Either way, there is increasing interest in combining cognitive-behavioral therapy with treatments known to reduce body weight. This topic is addressed more fully in Part II and Appendix II.

OTHER PSYCHOLOGICAL TREATMENTS

Many people who seek treatment for binge eating problems are veterans of one or more unsuccessful attempts to help them. This is often because the form of treatment offered was not optimal—not all forms of treatment help people with binge eating problems. Also, as mentioned, what works for some individuals does not work for others.

Despite the fact that no treatment appears to be as effective as cognitive-behavioral therapy, certain other psychological treatments have been shown to help some people.

Behavior Therapy

Two forms of behavior therapy have been studied, a treatment called *exposure with response prevention* and a simplified form of cognitive-behavioral therapy.

Exposure with Response Prevention. Devised by Drs. James Rosen and Harold Leitenberg of the University of Vermont, this form of treatment is designed for people who vomit after they binge. In its most typical form it involves getting people to binge to the point at which they would ordinarily vomit and then helping them resist doing so. Sessions of this therapy may last several hours.

Not surprisingly, patients usually do not like this treatment. The urge to vomit after binge eating is extremely strong, and resisting it is very distressing. The proponents of the treatment argue that self-induced vomiting is a major factor in keeping binge eating going; in support of this notion they point out that people with bulimia nervosa who know they are not going to be able to vomit more often than not are able to resist the urge to binge. Regardless of that and of the fact that vomiting certainly does worsen binge eating problems, exposure with response prevention has little to commend it. It is aversive, time-consuming, and not as effective as cognitive-behavioral therapy. On the other hand, it may have a role in helping those who do not benefit from cognitive-behavioral therapy.

Simplified Cognitive-Behavioral Therapy. This approach to treatment concentrates mainly on improving eating habits. It consists of the behavioral and educational components of cognitive-behavioral therapy but not the more technically demanding cognitive elements, so it is simpler to administer than the cognitive-behavioral treatment. This means it is suitable for use by less highly trained therapists. The research evidence to date suggests that it is not as effective as cognitive-behavioral therapy, since relapse tends to occur after the end of treatment. Nevertheless, this form of treatment is sufficient for some people. And this is an important point: Not everyone needs the full cognitive-behavioral treatment.

Psychoeducational Treatments

Psychoeducational treatment programs, usually conducted in a group setting, concentrate on educating people about binge eating problems and what they need to do to overcome them. The advice is usually based on that used in cognitive-behavioral therapy (for details, see Part II).

Researchers from Toronto studied the effectiveness of a form of this treatment that was unusual in that it was administered in a lecture format (see box opposite for details). They found that the psychoeducational treatment achieved results comparable to those obtained with cognitive-behavioral therapy except for those patients with more severe eating problems. Unfortunately, maintenance of change was not studied adequately, so the true benefits of this approach are not clear. Still, this finding reinforces the view that simpler treatments than cognitive-behavioral therapy are likely to be effective for a good number of those with binge eating problems.

Focal Psychotherapy

The term *focal psychotherapy* is generally used to refer to those brief forms of psychotherapy that first identify one or more issues that seem central to the patient's problem and then focus exclusively

Education as a Treatment for Bulimia Nervosa

Researchers in Toronto developed a brief educational treatment for bulimia nervosa. It consisted of five 90-minute lectures given over a 4-week period. (There were two lectures in the first week.) The lectures were accompanied by slides and were given classroom-style with chairs facing forward. Participants were encouraged to ask questions, but they were not asked to reveal personal information.

The lectures involved providing educational material and advice on how to overcome the eating problem. (This information and advice was similar to that provided in Part II of this book.) There was no personal guidance or support. The following topics were covered:

- The relationship between dieting and binge eating
- Body weight regulation
- The need to normalize food intake (i.e., stop dieting)
- Coping with urges to binge
- The adverse effects of self-induced vomiting, laxatives, and diuretics
- The need to stop vomiting and misusing laxatives and diuretics
- Myths about food and eating
- Common problematic attitudes toward food, eating, shape, and weight
- Social pressures on women to be thin
- The negative effects of evaluating self-worth in terms of shape and weight

The participants were encouraged to make changes on the basis of the information presented and to continue doing so after the end of the program.

The program was evaluated by comparing its effects with those obtained with cognitive-behavioral therapy conducted on a one-to-one basis. The two treatments were found to be equally effective, except for those people with more severe eating problems for whom one-to-one cognitive-behavioral therapy was superior.

This study is important since it indicates that sound information and advice on their own are sufficient to help many people with bulimia nervosa. The same is likely to be true for all those with binge eating problems.

Source: Olmsted MP, Davis R, Rockert W, Irvine M, Eagle M, Garner DM. Efficacy of a brief group psychoeducational intervention for bulimia nervosa. *Behaviour Research and Therapy* 1991; *29*: 71–83.

on the resolution of these problems. It is the intensity of their focus that characterizes them.

Interpersonal psychotherapy is one of the best-researched forms of focal psychotherapy. Devised originally to treat depression, it focuses on identifying and modifying those interpersonal problems thought to be responsible for episodes of depression—unresolved grief, disputes with friends or relatives, difficulties forming or maintaining relationships, and problems coping with life transitions (for example, leaving home, getting married, becoming a parent, among others).

Since interpersonal difficulties are common among those with binge eating problems (see Chapter 4) and may contribute to their maintenance (see Chapter 6), it is reasonable to expect this type of treatment to be helpful. To date only two studies of its use with binge eating problems have been conducted, however, although others are in progress. The first, a study from my group in Oxford, compared it with cognitive-behavioral therapy and behavior therapy in the treatment of bulimia nervosa and found it to be the least effective of the three at the end of treatment. However, the focal psychotherapy "caught up" and was as effective as cognitive-behavioral therapy twelve months and six years later, whereas, as already mentioned, patients who received behavior therapy had a tendency to relapse. This finding suggests that interpersonal psychotherapy may have a delayed effect but one that is still as powerful as that of cognitive-behavioral therapy. Interestingly, researchers from Stanford have found a group treatment based on interpersonal psychotherapy to be a promising treatment for binge eating disorder although the changes were not well maintained.

Group Therapy

For several reasons group therapy might be a good way of helping people with binge eating problems: It can dispel an individual's notion that he or she is the only one with this type of problem, which can be a great help. It can provide a venue through which members can learn from each other, as long as the group is run properly. And it makes practical sense, since much of the education and advice needed to help people with binge eating problems is suitable for presentation in a standardized form.

Unfortunately, until a direct comparison of group and individual versions of the same form of treatment is made, we will not be certain of the relative effectiveness of group and individual therapy. So far the research suggests that group therapy is somewhat less effective. Further, some people find the prospect of group therapy intolerable: They are so sensitive about their problem that they cannot consider the possibility of being treated in the presence of others.

Twelve-step programs, a type of group treatment, were discussed in Chapter 7.

Combined Psychological and Drug Treatment

Three studies have examined whether any advantage comes from using cognitive-behavioral therapy and antidepressant drugs in combination. Their results indicate that the combination has little to recommend it.

"STEPPED CARE" AND SELF-HELP

What does all the research mean to people with binge eating problems? If you or someone you know is seeking professional help, the implications are clear. The treatment of choice is cognitive-behavioral therapy on a one-to-one basis. Most people benefit substantially, and in the majority of cases the changes appear to last. It is important to understand, however, that some people do not improve or make only limited gains. For them additional treatment is needed. On the other hand, others respond to simpler forms of treatment involving education and advice.

Recently I proposed that a stepped-care treatment approach be adopted since it makes the best use of expertise and resources and spares people from undergoing unnecessary individual treatment. The approach involves offering a simple treatment first, because there are grounds for thinking that a significant number of people will respond. Only those who do not benefit move on to the next step involving a more intensive treatment. Again, a significant number will be expected to respond. Those who do not respond move on to the next step; and so on.

What should the steps be? It is my view that self-help would be the most appropriate first step for many people (see Figure 15), especially since it can be used in the absence of professional treatment. As Chapter 3 discussed, many people with binge eating problems are reluctant to seek outside help with their problem, so self-help is the ideal path for them. A suitable program forms Part II of this book.

Anyone who is unsuccessful in acting as his or her own therapist, or who doesn't want to, can move on to step 2 of the stepped-care program, what I call *guided self-help*. This involves following a self-help program with the support and guidance of a therapist. This therapist need not necessarily be a specialist in treating eating problems. Research from London and Cambridge suggests that this can work well. The program in Part II can be used in this way too.

The third step, should self-help prove insufficient, is the full cognitive-behavioral approach conducted on a one-to-one basis. Here a specialist is needed. More uncertain is what should follow

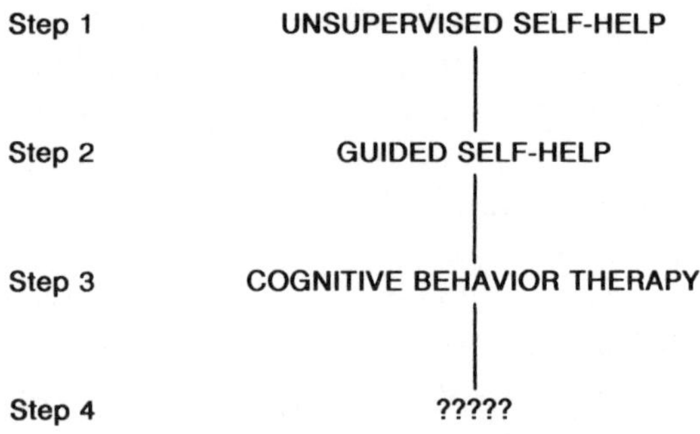

Figure 15. A stepped-care program.

if further treatment is required. Possibilities include focal psychotherapy, antidepressant drug treatment, and partial or full hospitalization. At present, there are no research findings to indicate which would be best. The decision therefore depends on the preferences of the patient and therapist and what treatment resources are available.

PART II

A SELF-HELP PROGRAM FOR THOSE WHO BINGE

Introduction

I READ THE PROGRAM from beginning to end and knew immediately that it made so much sense. I underlined point after point. It didn't simply say "Eat this" and "Avoid that." Rather, it explained how to get on the right track in a realistic step-by-step way. I felt inspired because it understood my problem. It was exactly what I was looking for and exactly what I needed.

For many years I have been studying the epidemiology, etiology, and treatment of binge eating problems. What became clear as early as 1980 was that few people with such problems seek outside help in solving them. I have watched that situation continue unchanged into the 1990s: As discussed in Part I, only 10 percent of those with bulimia nervosa are in treatment. This is not because they do not want help—far from it. The great majority would like to change, but, as discussed in Chapter 3, various barriers stand in their way. For more than ten years I have been convinced that self-help could provide an acceptable and accessible form of treatment—a way to surmount many of those barriers. What remained to be found was a therapy with proven lasting benefits that could be translated into a self-help format.

These two criteria ultimately converged in what my ongoing clinical studies had shown was by far the most effective treatment for binge eating problems: cognitive-behavioral therapy (see Chapter 8). After more than fifteen years of research, I was convinced that this approach did indeed have long-term benefits. That cognitive-behavioral therapy could be translated into a self-help format was also clear, thanks to the work of my colleague Dr. Peter Cooper, who reported that his adaptation of my cognitive-behavioral treatment for bulimia nervosa not only markedly reduced the necessary treatment time but also was popular and effective with his patients at Cambridge (see Further Reading).

This book and the self-help program here in Part II represent an extension of Dr. Cooper's work, in both focus and scale. This program is designed for all those who binge, including those with bulimia nervosa.

Of course no self-help program will be successful unless the person undertaking it sincerely wants to change. So if you or someone you know wishes to stop binge eating, it is imperative to begin with the following key section. *Do not proceed directly to Step 1 of the program.*

WHY CHANGE?

> *As I grow into middle age I realize with great sadness how much energy I have directed toward controlling my weight and eating and the misery of the regular and consequent binges. I could be doing something productive with my energy—building relationships, reading, writing. I don't know what I might do, but I don't want my epitaph to be "Jane wished she was thin." It was this, in the end, that made me decide to change.*

By this point in the book you should be sure, if you were not already, whether you binge. If you do binge, the key issue is whether you want to change. *Do you want to stop binge eating?* It is certainly possible to change: It is possible to start eating normally again; possible to enjoy eating rather than eat with fear, regret, or guilt; possible to be happy eating with others.

As discussed in Part I, how severely, if at all, binge eating affects a person's life varies greatly from individual to individual. Only you can decide how pressing the need is for change. But because your sense of urgency is very likely to waver, it often helps to have a set of guidelines by which you can measure the benefits of change unaffected by fluctuating daily circumstances. If you have a long history of binge eating, it is important that you examine how you have adjusted your life to accommodate your eating problem.

The Advantages

Start by drawing up a list of the potential advantages of change. To help you do so, ask yourself the following questions:

If I stop binge eating,

- Will I feel better about myself?
- Will it improve my quality of life?
- Will my physical health be enhanced?
- Will others benefit?

People are often surprised at how much better they feel once they stop binge eating. Even minor binge eating problems can have subtle adverse effects on many aspects of life. You may be unnecessarily irritable at times, your concentration may not be as good as it could be, you may avoid social events that you would really like to attend (see Chapter 4), and your physical health may be impaired (see Chapter 5). Perhaps you don't realize that these are direct results of your binge eating problem and will resolve as it improves. Another benefit of change is the effect it has on morale and self-image: Many people find it restores their sense of self-respect and self-worth. As mentioned in Chapter 4, one of the most gratifying aspects of helping people overcome binge eating problems is seeing the person underneath emerge as the problem recedes. The depression, tension, and irritability fade, concentration improves, and old interests (perhaps forgotten) return.

> *One of my difficulties in deciding to change was that it seemed self-indulgent. After all, lots of people have problems with their eating and weight. But the truth I had to face was that the problem was so much more invasive than it seemed—it affected everything. I couldn't be* me *while I still had the problem.*

Obviously one of the most compelling reasons to stop binge eating is the harm that the associated behaviors of dieting, self-induced vomiting, and laxative abuse may be doing to your health. When you stop doing these things, you can expect a gradual return of the normal sensations of fullness and hunger, an increase in energy, and an improvement in your overall sense of healthiness. As discussed in Chapter 5, binge eating and obesity are often associated, and while the exact relationship between the two is not fully understood, there is no doubt that you would be in a better position to control your weight if you had control over your eating. (To decide whether you are overweight and to learn how to adapt the program if you are, see Appendix II.)

The other people in your life—friends, family, and coworkers—will undoubtedly notice the blossoming of the person underneath as the binge eating problem recedes. You will stop being unpredictably irritable, touchy about eating and about your shape and weight, and sensitive about being with others. As a result, your relationships and your performance at work are bound to improve.

The Disadvantages

Of course, you should also consider possible disadvantages of change. There may be some, and it is worth balancing these against the advantages. You might be concerned about how you would feel if you did not succeed. Perhaps you are tempted to do nothing rather than risk failing. While this is understandable, it is a defeatist attitude that you should do your best to resist. There is every reason to expect that, with the right sort of help, your binge eating problem will improve. Furthermore, if you decide to use this self-help program and make a determined effort to do so, there can be no question of failure. *If things do not improve, the pro-*

gram simply was not right for you; it will have failed, not you. And if that is the case, many other options are available.

One other point to stress is that a good way of assessing the seriousness of a problem is to see how easy it is to overcome. If you discover that you can readily stop binge eating, then at least you have learned that the problem is surmountable. On the other hand, if you discover that it is not easy to change, you will have learned that it is a significant problem, perhaps more so than you thought. In this case you should perhaps consider taking it more seriously than you have been doing.

HOW TO CHANGE: THE VARIOUS OPTIONS

Assuming you have decided to tackle your binge eating problem, what should you do? The main options are described in Chapter 8. In principle you have four options:

1. *Seek professional help.* There are many professionals who help people who have eating problems. They include psychologists, psychiatrists, general physicians, dietitians, social workers, nurses, and others. Some specialize in the area. Information on how to find local specialists is given in Appendix III.
2. *Seek other forms of help.* For example, you could join a self-help group. Many such groups are excellent, but some are not. Some have questionable views on binge eating problems and how they should be tackled. Also, some are focused more on helping people live with their eating problem than on helping them overcome it. Before committing yourself to a self-help group, find out as much as you can about it through the agencies listed in Appendix III. If you do decide to join one, try it to see if it suits you. Remember, you can always leave if it isn't right for you.
3. *Use this self-help program.* Whether you are male or female,

single or married, living alone or with others, you can use this self-help program. You should reject this program only if one of the exclusion criteria in the box below applies to you.

4. *Combine professional help and self-help*. There are two ways to do this. You can use this self-help program on your own while at the same time receiving therapy of some other sort—therapy directed at, for example, self-esteem or relationships. This is a good plan so long as you have discussed it with your therapist. Therapists must be fully informed in case there is a clash between the program and the help they are providing.

   The other way of combining self-help and professional help is what may be called "guided self-help." This involves following the program with the support and guidance of a therapist. In this case the therapist acts as a supervisor who monitors progress, provides encouragement, and helps you identify potential solutions when you run into difficulties. The distinction between these two forms of self-help is discussed further in Appendix V.

Deciding What Is Best for You

If you think you need professional help, it is important that you take steps to obtain it. This self-help program must not divert you from doing so. On the other hand, this program, used with or without professional help, is likely to be appropriate for most people with binge eating problems. Therefore, it may well help you.

WHEN TO CHANGE

If you are thinking about changing but hesitate to commit yourself, I urge you to take the risk and get started. There is one point

When Self-Help May Not Help

You should not use this self-help program if any of the following exclusion criteria apply.

You are underweight. If your body mass index (see Appendix I) is below eighteen, your weight is definitely low. Table 8 shows what weights in pounds (for different heights) are equivalent to a body mass index of 18. If you weigh less than the weight shown for your height, you should use this program only under medical supervision, since it would be unwise for you to risk losing weight.

You have a serious physical illness. If you have a physical illness that might be affected by a change in your eating habits, you should use this program only under the supervision of a physician. This advice applies particularly to those with diabetes.

You are pregnant. Women who are pregnant should not use the program without first discussing the matter with their obstetrician.

Your physical health is being affected by the binge eating problem (see Chapter 5). If this applies, you should consult a physician to have your health checked before embarking on this program. Once you have done so and have received any necessary treatment, you may be in a position to use the program.

You are significantly depressed or demoralized. If you are feeling this way, you may not be able to summon up sufficient motivation to change. In this case you are unlikely to be able to make full use of the program. Instead you need to seek the advice of a professional regarding your feelings of depression. Once these feelings have lessened in severity, they may no longer interfere with your ability to follow the program, and you might well benefit from it.

You have general problems with impulse control (see Chapter 4). If, in addition to the problem with binge eating, you have problems with alcohol, drugs, or repeated self-harm, it would be best to seek professional help since this program on its own is unlikely to be sufficient.

Table 8. Are You Underweight?

Below is a list of weights for various different heights. These represent a body mass index of 18 (see Appendix I for an explanation). They apply to men and women. To determine whether you are underweight, find your height on the table and look across at the weight for that height. If you weigh less than this, your body mass index is below 18 and you have an unusually low weight. If you weigh more this, do *not* assume that you are overweight. To determine whether you are overweight, see Table 9 on page 208.

Height[a] (feet, inches)	Weight[b] (pounds)	Height[a] (feet, inches)	Weight[b] (pounds)
4'10"	86	5'8"	118
4'10½"	88	5'8½"	120
4'11"	89	5'9"	121
4'11½"	90	5'9½"	124
5'0"	91	5'10"	125
5'½"	93	5'10½"	127
5'1"	95	5'11"	128
5'1½"	96	5'11½"	131
5'2"	99	6'0"	132
5'2½"	100	6'½"	134
5'3"	101	6'1"	135
5'3½"	103	6'1½"	138
5'4"	105	6'2"	140
5'4½"	106	6'2½"	141
5'5"	108	6'3"	144
5'5½"	109	6'3½"	146
5'6"	112	6'4"	147
5'6½"	113	6'4½"	149
5'7"	114	6'5"	152
5'7½"	117	6'5½"	154

[a]Without shoes
[b]Without shoes, light indoor clothing

to note, however, and it applies to most forms of help but especially to this program: *It is best not to start until your chances of success are optimal.* If you are about to relocate, change jobs, get married, have a baby, or go on vacation, it is wise to delay starting for a few weeks or months. To get the most out of the program you will need at least a couple of months free from significant distractions. Anything less will not be enough.

WHAT TO CHANGE

There is one other important point to consider: your goals and how they match those of the program.

The primary goal of this program is to help you eat in a healthy fashion without binge eating. If you are to make a full and lasting recovery, you will need to eat at regular intervals through the day, you will need to eat adequate amounts of food, and you will need to make sure you are not avoiding any foods. How to achieve these goals is discussed in detail in the program.

What if your goals differ from those of this program? Perhaps, for example, your primary goal is to lose weight. In that case you may discover that there is a clash between what you want to achieve and the advice and information given here. Think carefully about doing things your way. After all, how well have these goals served you so far? Years of clinical experience and research inform this program and indicate that some things are just not possible. For instance, for many people most forms of dieting are simply incompatible with overcoming their binge eating problem since dieting makes them prone to binge.

Overcoming binge eating problems is not easy; it generally requires a lot of effort. Half-hearted attempts to change are unlikely to succeed. Give this program the benefit of the doubt by suspending your reservations and trying your best to make a fresh start.

HOW TO USE THE PROGRAM

The self-help program consists of six steps designed to be followed in the order specified (see box on page 140). As in the cognitive-behavioral treatment on which the program is based, the steps are additive; that is, each successive step involves adding

The Six Steps

Step 1. Getting started
Step 2. Regular eating
Step 3. Alternatives to binge eating
Step 4. Problem-solving and taking stock
Step 5. Dieting and related forms of avoidance
Step 6. What next?

something to what you have already been doing in the preceding step(s). It is not a good idea to dip around in the program, doing bits of this and bits of that. Start at the beginning and work your way through to the end, following the guidelines provided.

That said, be aware that not all the components of the program will be relevant to you. The program has been designed for all those who binge eat. As described in Part I, people who binge vary. The severity of the eating problem varies as does the presence of associated problems (see Chapter 4). Most people who binge also diet, often strictly, but some do not diet at all. Similarly, some are highly concerned about their appearance and weight, while others are not. Some are perfectionists and highly organized, whereas others are chaotic. Some are overweight; some are not. And some vomit or take laxatives or diuretics; others don't. All these features are relevant to binge eating and need to be addressed by the program. Therefore the program has many components, some of which will not apply to you. For the most part it will be obvious what applies and what does not. But when you are in doubt, the best policy is to assume that the advice does apply and follow it.

Here are some tips to help you succeed:

Persevere, especially when the advice seems difficult to follow. Often following the advice given in this program will be difficult, because it involves directly tackling the things that keep the binge eating problem going. In general, the harder you find it to follow the advice, the more important it is that you make your best effort to do so. Following the advice is the only way you will break out of the vicious circles that are maintaining your binge eating problem (see Chapters 4 and 6). However, keep in mind that *you will not need to follow the advice forever.* You will need to do many things to bring about change, but only some are relevant to ensuring that the changes persist in the future. These are discussed in Step 6.

Do not rush through the program. Instead, proceed at the pace suggested, since experience indicates that this will work best. Sometimes it is a good idea to stay at a step for an extra week or so to see if there is more that you can do. If you have a setback, it is often wise to go back a step.

In general, it takes people with longstanding binge eating problems between four and six months to work through the program and get the most out of it. Some people are able to change rapidly; for others it is a slow process. The key issue is whether you are making progress. If you are moving in the right direction, it is reasonable to carry on. On the other hand, if you have not benefited at all by the time you have reached Step 4, you should seek outside help. The same applies if you get stuck permanently.

Do not expect overnight success. Don't be disappointed by less-than-dramatic results. Change takes time, and binge eating problems are not likely to be resolved within just a few weeks.

Do not expect to make smooth and steady progress. It is normal for progress to occur in fits and starts. There are likely to be periods when things go well, times when you get stuck, and times when you have setbacks and the problem seems to worsen. In the course of the program, you will be monitoring your progress. This will allow you to identify and then tackle the obstacles that are interfering with your overcoming the problem.

Expect the urge to binge to persist. Even after you have completely stopped binge eating, the urge to binge often persists for several months. Don't be discouraged by this. The urge will be triggered by the same circumstances that used to trigger actual binges. This self-help program will help you resist this urge, and gradually it will fade away and disappear.

Be sure to hold review sessions. Until your binge eating is well under control, have two review sessions a week. Thereafter they can be weekly. It is a good idea to book them in advance and view them as equivalent to an appointment with a therapist, but in this case *you* are your own therapist. Try to set side fifteen to thirty minutes for these sessions. They are an important part of the program, and you should not allow other activities to take precedence over them.

Consider enlisting someone to help. While many people use the program on their own, others decide to enlist outside help. Such helpers fall into two categories, and their roles differ. You might choose a friend or relative, whose main role will be to provide support and encouragement at times of difficulty. Helpers of this type need to remain in the background unless their help is requested. In addition, or as an alternative, you may choose to seek the help of an independent therapist with whom you have a professional rather than personal relationship. Therapists can take a much more active role than friends or relatives. Indeed they can supervise your use of the program ("guided self-help"). Both groups of helpers need to be familiar with the program. (Appendix IV provides guidelines for relatives and friends, and Appendix V is for therapists.)

WHAT WILL HAPPEN TO YOUR WEIGHT?

Most people with binge eating problems are highly concerned about their appearance and weight, as Chapter 4 explained. Therefore, they want to know what will happen to their weight if they embark on the program. As discussed in Chapter 5, *generally there is little or no change in weight with recovery.* However, some people do gain weight and some lose, and it is impossible to predict what will happen in any individual case.

Thus it is not possible to give a precise answer to the question "What will happen to my weight?" If your weight is low as a result of your own efforts, you are likely to need to gain some weight. This is because continuing to diet is rarely compatible with overcoming a binge eating problem (with the possible exception of binge eating disorder). If this applies in your case, you have no other choice if you want to stop binge eating. On the other hand, if you are overweight (you have a body mass index over 27; see Table 9 in Appendix II), what will happen to your weight is less easy to predict, although I can say that you are most unlikely to gain weight. Specific advice for those who are overweight is provided in Appendix II.

At this stage *the best plan is for you to concentrate your efforts on overcoming the binge eating problem and to accept for the meantime whatever changes in weight occur.* Unless you have a general tendency to overeat (see Chapter 4), your weight will gradually move toward its natural level, which may be lower than, higher than, or much the same as its current level. And the truth is that it would be best for you to try to learn to live with this weight, since fighting it will mean an endless battle against your biology, a battle that unfortunately you can never win.

This may be difficult advice to accept, but following it is necessary if you are to overcome the problem. If this advice is unacceptable, try to suspend the question of your weight for, say, a month. At that point you can evaluate your progress in terms of your eating and weight and make an informed decision on whether you wish to continue. It is, of course, appropriate for you to monitor your weight as you work your way through the program. Advice on how to do so is given in Step 1.

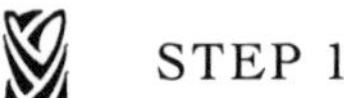

STEP 1

Getting Started

Step 1: Getting Started
Self-monitoring Weekly weighing

Step 2: Regular Eating
Establishing a pattern of regular eating Stopping vomiting and misusing laxatives and diuretics

Step 3: Alternatives to Binge Eating
Substituting alternative activities

Step 4: Problem Solving and Taking Stock
Practicing problem solving Reviewing progress

Step 5: Dieting and Related Forms of Avoidance
Tackling the three forms of dieting Tackling other forms of avoidance of eating

Step 6: What Next?
Preventing relapse Dealing with other problems

NOW THAT YOU ARE READY to start, the first thing you should do is familiarize yourself with the program. Quickly read through the rest of Part II so you get an overall picture of what lies ahead. Once you've done this, you are ready to start Step 1. It has two components, self-monitoring and weekly weighing.

SELF-MONITORING

Self-monitoring is central to this program. It serves two essential purposes:

1. Monitoring provides you with important information about your eating problem. You may say that you are all too aware of the problem. In a sense, of course, this is true. But accurate monitoring almost always highlights features that were not obvious beforehand. Monitoring gives you answers to these questions:

- Exactly what do you eat during your binges? How does it compare with what you eat at other times? Do your binges consist of foods that you are trying to avoid eating?
- Exactly when do your binges occur? Is there a predictable pattern? For example, do they always occur in the evening? Are weekdays any different from weekends?
- Are there any triggers for your binges? Do your binges tend to occur under certain circumstances? Do they occur when you are bored, depressed, lonely, or anxious?
- Do your binges appear to serve any function? For example, do they release feelings of tension? Are they a way of punishing yourself?

For reasons that will be explained later, you need the answers to these questions to overcome your binge eating problem.

2. Monitoring helps you change. When done properly, monitoring opens up possibilities for change. Monitoring your eating accurately and at the time you are doing it gradually reveals that apparently automatic, out-of-control behavior is nothing of the sort. You do not have to binge whenever you feel tense or angry or whenever you break one of your dietary rules. It is just that you have grown so used to doing so that doing anything else *seems* impossible. Monitoring along the lines recommended will show you that you have options other than binge eating. In this way it will help you change.

Why You Should Monitor—Despite Any Objections

At this stage you may find yourself reluctant to entertain the idea of monitoring. Perhaps you are already raising one of these objections:

- You have kept food records before, and it has not helped. In fact it is most unlikely that you have monitored in the way I recommend in this program. Keep an open mind.
- Monitoring sounds like too great a chore. You might feel that you are too busy or that your lifestyle makes it impossible. It is certainly true that monitoring is difficult for some people, but I have never encountered anyone whose lifestyle made it truly impossible for him or her to monitor. Your willingness to monitor is one test of your commitment to change.
- The shame you feel over your eating makes you unable to confront the problem in this way. If you feel like this, monitoring may indeed be particularly difficult. Nevertheless, if you are to overcome your binge eating problem, you have no alternative but to face up to it.
- You feel that monitoring will make you even more preoccupied with your eating than you already are. To an extent this may be true, but the preoccupation will be more constructive because it will be focused on how to overcome the eating problem.

How to Use the Monitoring Records

A blank monitoring record is shown as Figure 16. You may photocopy it or produce your own version modeled on it. You'll need a fresh record for each day, and you'll need to carry it with you wherever you go.

Figure 17 shows a monitoring record completed by a woman with binge eating disorder. You can see that during her evening meal she ate more potato salad than she had intended and that soon afterward a binge started, the trigger being her decision to give up controlling her eating.

Day . . . . Date . . . .

Time	Food and drink consumed	Place	*	V/L	Context and comments

Figure 16. A blank monitoring record. (See instructions on p. 148.) Permission to reproduce this form is granted to purchasers of *Overcoming Binge Eating* for personal use only.

Instructions for the Monitoring Record (see Figure 16)

Column 1: Note the time when you eat or drink anything. Do your best to be accurate.

Column 2: Record exactly what you eat and drink, including binges. Leave nothing out. Do not record calories. Instead, write down a simple description of what you eat and drink. Write down each item as soon as possible after you eat it. Trying to recall what you ate or drank some hours earlier is not a good idea since it is unreliable and will not help you change. The importance of monitoring *at the time of eating* cannot be overemphasized. For example, if you are out for a meal, it is sometimes sensible to record between courses, perhaps by going to the bathroom to get some privacy. Only in this way will monitoring help you change.

Episodes of eating that you view as meals should be identified with brackets. Do not bracket snacks or other episodes of eating.

Column 3: Specify where you consumed the food or drink. If in your home, specify the room.

Column 4: Place an asterisk in this column opposite the food items that you felt at the time were excessive. Binges will therefore be represented by a chain of asterisks.

Column 5: Record if and when you vomit or misuse laxatives or diuretics.

Column 6: Use this column somewhat like a diary. You should note anything that influences your eating. For example, whenever you put an asterisk in column 4, you should record in column 6 the circumstances at the time to identify triggers for the episode of excessive eating. Perhaps you had just had an argument with someone and were angry. Or you may have been under social pressure to eat.

Also use column 6 to record your weight each time you weigh yourself.

What You Should Do

Start monitoring as just described, but don't try to change your eating. It is important to start by getting into the habit of accurate monitoring. You will be changing your eating in Step 2. Monitoring must become a habit since you will be doing it for the duration of the program. Don't take days off from monitoring (or from the program) and don't omit binges from your record. *This may be difficult, but it is essential to be honest with yourself.*

Keep your monitoring records somewhere private and keep them together so that you can look back over them. This will allow you to detect trends over time and thereby assess the extent to which you have changed. (If you are taking the guided self-

Day Saturday Date September 27

Time	Food and drink consumed	Place	*	V/L	Context and comments
8:10	1 plain bagel 1 cup decaf	Office			Feel good. Determined to do well.
8:25	1 cup decaf	Office			
11:00	1 banana	Office			
1:10	1 cup vegetable soup Small vanilla yogurt	Office – at desk			
8:00	Pasta salad with salami Potato salad	Kitchen	*		Too much – I've broken my diet yet again.
8:20	6 scoops ice cream 10-15 Ritz crackers 16 oz bag potato chips Diet coke Large slice chocolate cake 5 KitKats Diet coke	Kitchen	* * * * *		Crying. Feel my life is pointless. I can't stop. I've no self-control. I just give up.
9:50	Diet coke	Bedroom			
10:30	Diet coke	Bedroom			

Figure 17. A completed monitoring record.

help approach, you will need to review your monitoring records with your therapist.)

So, begin by monitoring until your first review session in three or four days.

WEEKLY WEIGHING

Most people with binge eating problems are concerned about their weight, and often this is a major concern. Weighing may therefore be very important to them. As described in Chapter 4, many go through a period of weighing themselves very frequently, in some cases many times a day. However, weighing as often as this can become intolerable, and consequently some switch to not weighing themselves at all while remaining highly concerned about their weight.

As a result of following this program, it is highly likely that your eating habits will change. It is therefore appropriate that you monitor your weight. The best way of doing this is to weigh yourself once a week. To identify changes in your weight, don't rely too heavily on individual readings since body weight fluctuates from day to day. Single readings can therefore be misleading. Instead, look for trends over several weeks (three or four readings) since only in this way can you detect true changes.

What You Should Do

Start weighing yourself once a week on a preset morning of your choice. A weekday is usually best since on weekends you may dwell on any changes that have occurred. Do your best not to weigh yourself between these times.

Many people find this difficult advice to follow. If you are used to weighing yourself more often than this, you may feel uneasy decreasing the frequency of weighing. You may be afraid that your weight will go up without your knowing. If you have been avoiding weighing, you may be afraid that restarting will lead you to become preoccupied with your weight and as a result you will want to weigh yourself more often than once a week. Whether this applies to you or not, do your best to stick to weighing yourself once a week. This way you will detect changes that occur without being distracted by day-to-day fluctuations.

You may need to buy a scale. An inexpensive bathroom scale is fine. And if you are tempted to weigh yourself between your weekly weighings, move the scale to a place where it is out of sight and relatively inaccessible so that the temptation is easier to resist.

REVIEWING STEP 1

This review session should focus on your monitoring and weighing after you have followed the Step 1 guidelines for three or four days. You will be having another review session after three or four more days on Step 1 (i.e., two review sessions a week).

Reread Step 1 to remind yourself what you were to do. Then ask yourself the following questions (see box below):

1. Have I been monitoring? If your answer is yes, you have made a good start. If your answer is no, you have a serious problem. Carefully consider your reasons for not monitoring, perhaps rereading the section on why monitoring is important. (It is a good idea, in fact, to reread the program at regular intervals. It contains a great deal of information, and it is difficult to absorb it

Review Checklist for Step 1

- Have I been monitoring?
- Can I improve my monitoring?
- Are any patterns in my eating becoming obvious?
- Am I weighing myself once a week?

all at one sitting. Also, some of the advice may not apply at first but will apply later on. It is especially important that you reread sections on which you get stuck or make limited or slow progress.)

Perhaps you should reconsider the advantages and disadvantages of change. If the advantages outweigh the disadvantages, you should make a fresh commitment to monitor. You are unlikely to make significant progress without monitoring. Remember, it provides you with important information and helps you change.

If you decide to make another attempt at monitoring, reread the section on how to monitor and examine your progress at the next review session.

2. Can I improve my monitoring? Study your monitoring records to see whether there is any room for improvement. Have you been following all the guidelines? For example, has your monitoring been accurate? Have you written things down as soon as possible after their consumption? Have you bracketed meals? Have you used the asterisks in the way described? Have you been writing in column 6?

3. Are any patterns in my eating becoming obvious? Have you had any binges? Do they have anything in common? Have they happened at the same time of day? What about their triggers? Can you identify them?

What have you eaten in your binges? Is there anything characteristic about the food? Why are you eating these particular foods? Are they foods you are avoiding at other times?

What are you eating outside your binges? Are you dieting or avoiding eating? Are you having normal meals?

Are all your days the same, or do they differ? Do you alternate between days on which you diet and days when you binge?

Try to answer these questions honestly. Doing so will increase your understanding of the problem and will highlight things that need to be changed.

4. Am I weighing myself once a week? If so, record the weight on your summary sheet (described in the next section). If not, work out what the problem is. If you are weighing yourself too often, devise a way of resisting doing that. Is your scale out of sight and relatively inaccessible? If you are not weighing yourself at all, you must find the courage to begin. Remember you are starting on this program to regain control over your eating and as you succeed your weight may change. It is much better to know what is really happening to your weight than to keep your head in the sand and fear the worst.

WHEN TO MOVE ON

Continue monitoring until your second review session in three or four days. Then review your monitoring following the preceding guidelines. Ask yourself the same four questions.

Next, start a summary sheet. A blank sheet is shown as Figure 18. Photocopy this one or make your own. You will be using the summary sheet to chart your progress as you go through the program.

Look at Figure 19, a partly completed summary sheet. It charts the progress of someone who is six weeks into the program.

Now look at your own summary sheet. How many good days did you have? If you had six or seven, you are ready to move on. In that case, read through Step 2 and follow its advice while continuing with Step 1 (monitoring and weekly weighing). If you had fewer than six or seven good days, try to identify why and continue with Step 1 until your next review session. Remember, it is important not to rush through the program. To get maximum benefit, you need to accomplish each step before moving on to the next.

Week	B	V/L/D	"GDs"	Wt	Events
1					
2					
3					
4					
5					
6					
7					
8					
9					
10					
11					
12					
13					
14					
15					
16					
17					
18					
19					
20					
21					
22					
23					
24					

Figure 18. A blank summary sheet. (See instructions, opposite.) Permission to reproduce this form is granted to purchasers of *Overcoming Binge Eating* for personal use only.

Instructions for the Summary Sheet (see Figure 18)

Column 1: This indicates how many weeks you have been following the program. You have now completed your first week.

Column 2: Record how many binges you had over the last seven days. You should get this figure from your monitoring records.

Column 3: Record the number of times you practiced any extreme method of weight control, such as self-induced vomiting or misusing laxatives or diuretics. Record each behavior separately. Again, you should get these figures from your monitoring records.

Column 4: Record how many "good days" (GDs) you had during the week. *A good day is one on which you did your best to change by following the program.* The definition of a good day will alter as you work through the program. At this point a good day is one on which you monitored accurately.

Column 5: Record your weight. If you weighed yourself more than once during the week, record the weight you were on the morning on which you were meant to weigh yourself.

Column 6: Record other points of note. For example, you should record when you move from one step of the program to the next. Also note any events that significantly influenced your eating; for example, being ill or away from home.

Week	B	V/L/D	"GDs"	Wt	Events
1	9		4	142	Started Step 1
2	7		7	144	
3	4		5	143	Step 2
4	3		5	139	
5	5		7	139	Got worse – Why?
6	2		5	140	Saw parents on weekend
7					
8					
9					
10					
11					
12					
13					
14					
15					
16					
17					
18					
19					
20					
21					
22					
23					
24					

Figure 19. A summary sheet from someone six weeks into the program.

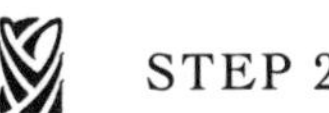

STEP 2

Regular Eating

Step 1: Getting Started
Self-monitoring
Weekly weighing

Step 2: Regular Eating
Establishing a pattern of regular eating
Stopping vomiting and misusing laxatives and diuretics

Step 3: Alternatives to Binge Eating
Substituting alternative activities

Step 4: Problem Solving and Taking Stock
Practicing problem solving
Reviewing progress

Step 5: Dieting and Related Forms of Avoidance
Tackling the three forms of dieting
Tackling other forms of avoidance of eating

Step 6: What Next?
Preventing relapse
Dealing with other problems

INTRODUCING A PATTERN of regular eating is probably the single most potent element in this program. It involves restricting your eating to three planned meals each day plus two or three planned snacks. *Introducing this pattern of regular eating displaces binges* with the result that their frequency progressively decreases. Binge eating that once was frequent now becomes intermittent.

HOW TO INTRODUCE A PATTERN OF REGULAR EATING

Your aim should be to eat three planned meals each day plus two or three planned snacks. A typical pattern would be:

8:00 A.M.: Breakfast
10:30 A.M.: Midmorning snack
12:30 P.M.: Lunch
3:30 P.M.: Midafternoon snack
7:00 P.M.: Evening meal
9:00 P.M.: Evening snack

At this stage in the program, when you eat should be dictated by your preset plan and not by sensations of hunger or other urges to eat. Popular articles often tell us to listen to our body's signals and eat in response to them. This apparently wholesome advice ignores the fact that these signals are often disturbed in those who binge. Erratic eating, especially when it consists of alternating binge eating and dieting, disrupts the normal mechanisms that control sensations of hunger and fullness, so these feelings are no longer a reliable guide for when to eat. Later, once you are eating regularly, without overeating and without dieting, normal sensations of hunger and fullness will gradually return. When this happens, you can use these sensations to guide your eating, although maintaining a pattern of regular eating should remain a priority.

If your eating is very chaotic, you may not be able to introduce this eating pattern all at once. In this case introduce it gradually, starting with the part of the day that is least chaotic. This is usually the morning. So, start by introducing breakfast and lunch (and possibly a midmorning snack) according to the guidelines given here. Then, over the next few weeks, gradually introduce the other meals and snacks until the full pattern is in place.

Leave no more than three to four hours between planned meals and snacks. Because morning is the least chaotic time for most people, you might be able to allow a longer interval at that time of day. You will need to adjust the exact timing of your meals and snacks to suit your commitments, but try to establish as regular a pattern as possible. The timing may need to vary from day to day; you will probably, for instance, want weekends to differ from weekdays.

Do not skip meals or snacks. This is important, because skipping a scheduled meal or snack will make you vulnerable to binge at these times.

Between the planned meals and snacks, do your best not to eat. In this way your day will be divided up by the meals and snacks. They will be like stepping-stones through the day. So, using our typical pattern, morning will be the time between breakfast and lunch, early afternoon will be the period between lunch and your midafternoon snack, late afternoon will be between your midafternoon snack and your evening meal, and the evening will be divided in two by your evening snack. Breaking periods of unstructured time into discrete units of no longer than three to four hours will help reduce the frequency of binge eating, since most people are prone to binge when faced with long periods of unstructured time.

If things go wrong and you eat (or binge) between meals and snacks, it is important to get back on track as rapidly as possible. Do your best to resist the temptation to avoid (or cut down the size of) your next meal or snack, since doing so will increase the risk of further problems.

Where possible, this pattern of eating should take precedence over other activities. Don't push it aside or forget it because of other priorities. Make every effort to leave room in your day for the meals and snacks, although occasionally they will need to be juggled to accommodate major commitments. For example, if for some reason you know that your evening meal will be late, say at 10:00 P.M., then a sensible plan would be to move the evening snack earlier to midway between the midafternoon snack and the 10:00 P.M. evening meal.

At the beginning of each day (or the preceding evening), work out when you are going to eat and write down the times at the top of your monitoring record (see page 162). At all points of the day you should know when you are next going to eat. If a particular day is so unpredictable that it is impossible to plan the entire day, plan ahead as far as you can and schedule a review time for when you will be in a position to plan the remainder of the day.

At this stage in the program, the focus is not on what you eat but on when you eat. It really does not matter at this stage what you consume in your meals and snacks. What is important is that you eat food that you are comfortable with. Make sure you have adequate supplies of such "safe" food available. If you are going to plan when to eat, you might ask, don't you have to plan what and how much to eat as well? You do not have to do this, but you can if you wish to. This is fine as long as it does not cause you too much anxiety.

It also helps to plan in advance—the night before or first thing in the morning—so that you are not left with any last-minute decisions to make.

Some people are tempted to eat very little in their meals or snacks for fear of gaining weight. This is not wise, since it can increase the risk of binge eating by creating physiological pressures to eat. Therefore, try not to eat too little. *And you certainly must not attempt to compensate for what you have eaten by vomiting or taking laxatives or diuretics.*

My general advice is to aim for a broad range of foods and average-sized portions. The size of an average portion can be determined from the eating habits of friends or relatives, from recipes, and from the notations on nondiet food packages. Or, if someone is helping you with the program, ask his or her advice on what is a reasonable amount to eat.

Adopting this pattern of regular eating may make you feel

full even after eating relatively little. This is particularly likely if you are not used to eating without subsequently vomiting or taking laxatives or diuretics. Such feelings may be exaggerated by wearing tight clothes. It is important for you to know that these feelings of fullness almost always subside within an hour or so. They are best dealt with by avoiding wearing tight clothes at mealtimes and by engaging in distracting activities afterward (explained in Step 3). As mentioned earlier, normal feelings of fullness will gradually return.

Do your best to stick to your plan and review your progress at the end of each day. Then make whatever adjustments seem appropriate. For example, you may discover that you are having your evening snack so late in the day that it is not breaking up the evening. In that case, try moving it to an earlier time.

Figure 20 shows a monitoring record completed by someone with bulimia nervosa who was at this stage in the program. You can see that at the top of the record she wrote down when she planned to eat and that, apart from dinner, she did well at sticking to her plan.

HOW YOUR WEIGHT WILL BE AFFECTED

You may be concerned that eating regular meals and snacks will make you gain weight. You are especially likely to have this concern if at present you diet strictly and eat few, if any, meals or snacks. You may say that you are already struggling with your weight and that introducing meals and snacks is bound to make your weight go up.

The effect of treatment on weight was discussed in Part I. In practice *introducing regular meals and snacks does not tend to result in weight gain.* Indeed, you can anticipate either no change in weight or some weight loss, because the frequency of binge eating drops as this pattern of eating displaces the binges. And since most binges contain a large number of calories, even a slight decline in

Breakfast – 8
Lunch – 12:30
Aft. snack – 3:30
Dinner – 7:00
Eve. snack – 9:00

Day ..Thursday....... Date ..June 4.........

Time	Food and drink consumed	Place	*	V/L	Context and comments
7:40	Orange juice				To tide me over until breakfast.
8:10	Bowl Bran Flakes Muffin – small Decaf	Kitchen			Mustn't eat too much since I'm late and tense about work.
12:35	Turkey sandwich Potato salad – small Apple Decaf	At work			Potato salad a little risky. Probably have had too large a lunch but it was planned.
3:15	Apple Diet coke	Work			
5:40	Apple juice	Kitchen			Thirsty – after run.
7:00	Large slice of pizza Ice cream – 2 scoops 1 decaf		*		Shouldn't have had ice cream. Eaten too much today.
9:10	Small piece of apple pie				Planned snack.

Figure 20. A monitoring record showing a pattern of regular eating.

their frequency will result in a significant drop in overall calorie intake. This applies even if the binges are followed by vomiting or taking laxatives or diuretics, since none of these methods gets rid of all the food that has been eaten. (If you have doubts about this, you might find it helpful to reread Chapters 4 and 5 to remind yourself about the ineffectiveness of these methods of weight control.)

SOME ADVICE ON MEALS

Meals can be a problem for those who binge. They can lead to trouble in a variety of ways. Some of the following suggestions may not be relevant to you or may not be applicable because of your circumstances. Nevertheless, read through them and try those that are relevant. *Keep in mind that you will not have to behave permanently in this way.* These are interim measures designed to help you regain control over eating, and you can drop them once you no longer need them.

Restrict eating to certain places in your home. Part of regaining control over eating involves formalizing it. It is a good idea to have one or two set places where you eat. These should be at a table or equivalent and should not be within arm's reach of supplies of food. You should not eat in your bedroom or in the bathroom. If you have only one room, I recommend that you restrict your eating to one place in the room.

Concentrate when eating. While it may be tempting to distract yourself when eating, this is not a good idea. Instead, it is important that you focus on what you are doing. You need to learn to savor food. You also need to check that you are not eating in an abnormal way. For example, it is important not to eat too fast. Being aware of what you are doing will also help ensure that your meals and snacks do not turn into binges. With this end in mind:

- *Do not engage in any other activity when eating* (such as watching television).
- *Sit down when eating.* Eating on the move can result in "grazing."

When eating, restrict the availability of food. When eating a meal or snack, have only a preplanned amount of food at hand. Whenever practicable, keep packages and serving dishes off the table in case you are tempted to eat more than you had intended.

Practice controlling your eating.

- *Practice putting down your utensils between mouthfuls.*
- *Insert a number of pauses in your meals.*
- *Practice leaving some food on the plate.* This may seem wasteful, but anything that will prevent you from binge eating is not truly wasteful.
- *Discard leftovers.* At this stage they may be too tempting.

When eating with others, do not be persuaded to eat more than you had planned. Many people are put under pressure to have second helpings or larger quantities than they want. You must resist this pressure. Practice polite but firm ways of refusing—e.g., "No, thank you. I have really had enough. It was delicious." If someone still puts unwanted food on your plate, leave it untouched. Under these circumstances it is really that person who is being impolite, not you.

When eating a meal out, take stock between courses. It is easy for meals in restaurants or at other people's homes to get out of hand. You may not know how many courses there will be or what they will contain. You therefore need to keep a careful eye on what is happening. To do so, make sure that you do not drink too much alcohol since this will impair your judgment and willpower. In meals with a large number of courses, it is often easier to skip one or two courses altogether than to try to limit the amount you eat at each course. Buffets are a particular challenge. The best approach is to look over what is offered and then plan what to eat.

SOME ADVICE ON SHOPPING AND COOKING

Many people with binge eating problems have difficulties with shopping and cooking, largely due to the ready availability of food. As with the advice concerning meals, not all of the following suggestions may be relevant to you.

Limit your stock of "dangerous" food. At this stage it is best to restrict the availability of foods that trigger your binges as well as foods on which you binge. Therefore, when shopping, avoid buying these foods. If this is not practical, limit the quantities that you buy.

Ensure that you have adequate supplies of "safe" food. It is important that you have stocks of food that you feel comfortable eating.

Plan your shopping. Do not shop for food on the spur of the moment. Instead, plan it in advance. If possible, avoid shopping on days when you feel at risk of binge eating. You may find it helpful to shop with a relative or friend.

Restrict the amount of money you carry. On days when you feel you might binge, it may be helpful to limit the amount of money you carry, thereby making it difficult to buy the necessary food.

When cooking, avoid tasting. Picking at what you're cooking can trigger binges. Some people find it helpful to chew gum since this makes picking almost impossible.

Avoid unnecessary exposure to food.

- *Cooking.* Many people with binge eating problems like to cook, and the preoccupation with food and eating that accompanies binge eating problems encourages their interest in food. Partly as a consequence, some spend a lot of time cooking for others. This is to be resisted since, for obvious reasons, unnecessary exposure to food is risky.

- *Working with food.* In some cases the advice to limit exposure to food has to be extended to working with food. It is not uncommon for those with binge eating problems to work directly or indirectly with food. For example, many work in restaurants or as nutritionists. If exposure to food is contributing significantly to your binge eating problem and is limiting your ability to overcome it, seriously consider changing your job.
- *Serving food.* Some people with binge eating problems have a tendency to press food on others. This is not a good idea. Instead, treat others as you would want to be treated. Offer them food, but do not pressure them to take some.

WHAT TO DO ABOUT SELF-INDUCED VOMITING

Some people with binge eating problems vomit after eating (see Chapter 4). In the great majority, this vomiting occurs only after binge eating. Therefore, if the frequency of binge eating falls, so will the frequency of vomiting. For this reason vomiting usually does not need to be tackled separately. The only appropriate advice is to choose meals and snacks that you are prepared not to get rid of; and if you are tempted to vomit after eating, do your best to resist the urge. Just as feelings of fullness decline after eating, so do urges to vomit. So, if you have a strong urge to vomit, distract yourself for a while and perhaps make vomiting more difficult by staying in the company of others. *Remember, vomiting encourages further binge eating.*

A small minority of people vomit after eating anything at all. If this applies to you and you are unable to stop, you should seek professional help. This is a difficult habit to overcome on your own.

WHAT TO DO ABOUT LAXATIVE AND DIURETIC MISUSE

As explained in Chapter 4, people with binge eating problems may misuse laxatives in two ways. They may take them to compensate for specific episodes of overeating, in which case the behavior is very similar to self-induced vomiting. Or they may take them on a regular basis, independent of particular episodes of overeating, in which case the behavior is more like dieting. Diuretics tend to be taken in the second way.

What was just said about self-induced vomiting applies equally to the first type of laxative misuse. On the other hand, if you are taking laxatives and diuretics regularly, my advice is simply to stop taking them. Perhaps surprisingly, most people find that they are able to do this simply by putting their mind to it, especially once they appreciate how ineffective these methods are at preventing calorie absorption (see page 52). *If you find that you are unable to stop, phase out the laxatives or diuretics by halving your daily consumption after each of your twice-a-week review sessions.*

It is important to remember that if you have been taking laxatives or diuretics frequently, stopping them suddenly can result in a period of fluid retention lasting a week or so, and obviously this is associated with some weight gain. If this happens, keep in mind that the gain in weight is temporary and will go away as the extra fluid is lost.

What You Should Do

Introduce the pattern of regular eating while continuing to monitor. Assess your progress at the next review session in three or four days.

Do not expect it to be easy to start eating in this way. You may well have problems. For example, you are likely to want to eat when you should not; conversely, you might not want to eat when you should. Do your best, at the same time noting down on your monitoring records any difficulties you are having. Many of the suggestions that have been made regarding meals, shopping and cooking should help you deal with these difficulties. Further suggestions are made in Steps 3 and 4.

REVIEWING STEP 2

It usually takes several weeks to establish this pattern of regular eating. As mentioned, mornings are often the easiest time of day. Therefore, if need be, start with the mornings and try to impose the pattern on them. Then, over the next few weeks, progressively move through the day, inserting the other meals and snacks.

To review your progress, study your monitoring records (see box below). As mentioned, doing so at the end of each day is a

Review Checklist for Step 2

- Can I improve my monitoring?
- Are any patterns in my eating becoming obvious?
- Am I weighing myself once a week?
- Each day, am I planning regular meals and snacks?
- Am I trying to restrict my eating to the day's meals and snacks?
- Am I skipping any of the meals and snacks?
- Are the gaps between my meals and snacks no longer than three to four hours?
- Am I eating between my meals and snacks?
- Am I getting back on track when things go wrong?
- Am I adjusting the timing of my meals and snacks to accommodate special situations?
- Am I following the advice regarding self-induced vomiting and the misuse of laxatives and diuretics?

good idea at this stage, but in addition you should continue to hold twice-a-week review sessions at which you examine your overall progress. *At the end of each full week, complete a summary sheet.* A "good day" at this stage is one on which you monitored accurately and did your best to stick to your planned pattern of eating, irrespective of whether or not you binged.

At the review sessions, ask yourself the following questions in addition to those from Step 1.

1. Each day, am I planning regular meals and snacks? Remember, this is central to the program. Indeed, you are unlikely to overcome your binge eating problem without following this advice. While I would not recommend that your eating always be this regimented, for the meantime it is important that you plan ahead. *To get control over your eating, you need to be one step ahead of the problem rather than one step behind it.* Each morning (or the previous evening if this suits you better) you should work out when you will be eating your next day's meals and snacks, and you should do your best to stick to this plan. This way you will be more likely to foresee problems than come upon them unawares.

2. Am I trying to restrict my eating to the day's meals and snacks? Again, this is central to the program.

3. Am I skipping any of the meals and snacks? It is important that you do not skip any meals or snacks since doing so will make you vulnerable to binge during the gaps.

4. Are the gaps between my meals and snacks no longer than three to four hours? For the same reason, the gaps between the meals and snacks should not be long, rarely longer than three to four hours.

5. Am I eating between my meals and snacks? The goal is to restrict your eating to the planned meals and snacks. If you are succeeding in doing this, your monitoring records will have an obvious clear pattern to them. Furthermore, this pattern should match the plan written at the top.

Almost certainly you will still be having binges at this stage.

Don't feel despondent about this. The important thing is that after each binge you try to get back on track as soon as possible. You must try hard not to skip the next meal or snack since this will only make you vulnerable to binge once again.

6. Am I getting back on track when things go wrong? It is important not to give up whenever something goes wrong. There is a tendency for people with binge eating problems to view days as a single unit, with the result that when anything goes wrong they write off the whole day as ruined. This is not helpful and is an example of all-or-nothing thinking (see Chapter 4). You must do your best to return to your plan as soon as possible rather than wait until the next day before restarting.

7. Am I adjusting the timing of my meals and snacks to accommodate special situations? Your eating pattern must not be too rigid, or you will run into difficulties when faced with special situations such as meals out, vacations, and holidays. Examine your monitoring records to see whether there have been any such circumstances and see how you have dealt with them.

8. Am I following the advice regarding self-induced vomiting and the misuse of laxatives and diuretics? All three of these extreme weight control behaviors encourage binge eating. It is essential that you stop them by following the guidelines provided.

WHEN TO MOVE ON

Most people need to spend several weeks at this stage. However, *you do not need to wait until you are having seven good days each week before moving on, because Step 3 will help you follow Step 2.* What is essential is that you are able to give the appropriate answer to all eight of the review questions. If you cannot, then you should reread Step 2 and stay at this stage for at least another week.

If you are ready to move on, continue with Steps 1 and 2 while starting to implement Step 3.

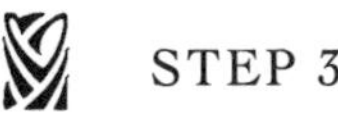 STEP 3

Alternatives to Binge Eating

Step 1: Getting Started
Self-monitoring Weekly weighing

Step 2: Regular Eating
Establishing a pattern of regular eating Stopping vomiting and misusing laxatives and diuretics

Step 3: Alternatives to Binge Eating
Substituting alternative activities

Step 4: Problem Solving and Taking Stock
Practicing problem solving Reviewing progress

Step 5: Dieting and Related Forms of Avoidance
Tackling the three forms of dieting Tackling other forms of avoidance of eating

Step 6: What Next?
Preventing relapse Dealing with other problems

AN IMPORTANT SKILL TO DEVELOP is the ability to resist urges to binge. At Step 2 you were trying to confine your eating to planned meals and snacks. While some people have little difficulty doing this, others have problems. To help you avoid eating between your planned meals and snacks, you will find it useful to have a range of alternative activities.

HOW TO USE ALTERNATIVE ACTIVITIES

Construct a list of alternative activities. You need to think of all those activities that are either incompatible with eating or make eating very difficult. These will differ from person to person, but here are some typical examples:

- Exercising, e.g., swimming, brisk walking, cycling, jogging, aerobics.
- Going out with the children.
- Taking a shower or bath.
- Visiting or calling certain friends or relatives, especially anyone who is helping you with this program.
- Playing music. (Some people find they cannot binge when certain types of music are playing. They say the atmosphere is just not right.)

You need to devise a list that is appropriate for you. In general, the activities need to be active (i.e., involve doing something) rather than passive (such as watching television). Also, they should not feel like a chore; rather, they should be enjoyable.

Write down the list of alternative activities on a small card and carry it around with you. This list should be available for use at difficult times.

When you have an urge to eat between your planned meals and snacks, immediately note this down in column 6 of your monitoring record. Then take out your list of activities and work through them one by one. Say it is 7:00 P.M., and you have eaten your evening meal. Perhaps you feel that you ate too much and you are tempted to give in and binge. Perhaps you are also tired, having had a stressful day, and you have nothing planned for the evening. Clearly you are at risk. Now, if you are recording properly, you will be well aware that a potential problem is looming. You will be one step ahead of the problem. You will have written down your evening meal and also something in column 6 along the following lines: "Feel as if I've eaten too much. I'm tired, and there's a long evening ahead of me. Strong urge to binge." What should you do under these circumstances?

There are two related problems here. The first is your urge to binge, and the second is the fact that you have nothing to do. This step of the program will focus on the first of these problems, dealing with the urge to binge. Step 4 will address the second.

Three things should happen if you are to deal successfully with the urge to binge:

1. Time must pass. Urges to binge fade with time. Even half an hour may be long enough for the urge to decline sufficiently for you to resist it easily. So, you need to engage in something distracting for a while.
2. You must make it difficult for you to binge.
3. You must do something else, preferably something that is pleasurable.

So, get out your list of alternative activities and review it. It is 7:00 P.M., and you have no plans for the evening. What should you do? You decide to do two things. First, you decide to exercise since, although you don't feel in the mood, you know that you will feel better for having done so and you will not be tempted to eat while exercising. Also, exercising will help you unwind. But, before starting to exercise, you also decide to call some friends to see if someone is free later on to meet for coffee. So, first you call friends on your list of alternative activities to see if it is possible to meet later, and then you exercise, followed by a shower. And all the time you are aware that you are due to have your evening snack at around 9:00 P.M.

With a plan like this it is likely that you will be able to resist the urge to binge. Calling friends will be distracting and, with any luck, will give you something to do later on. Exercising and then taking a shower will occupy time and will make you feel better about yourself.

You may find that at first the urge to binge takes quite a while to subside and disappear. However, you will notice that the urge fades more and more quickly as you practice engaging in alternative activities. Eventually it will disappear altogether or be so weak that you can easily ignore it.

A negative effect of resisting eating between your planned meals and snacks is also worth mentioning. Namely, the unpleasant feelings and thoughts that trigger some binges will no longer be blocked out. As a result some people feel worse at times despite the lift in mood that comes from bingeing less often. Step 4 discusses how to deal with these triggers.

What You Should Do

You need to practice engaging in alternative activities when you have the urge to eat between your planned meals and snacks. Sometimes you will not succeed; sometimes you will. With practice it will become progressively easier. Assess your progress at each of your twice-a-week review sessions.

There are two general goals: First, you need to become good at spotting urges to binge as early as possible. Second, you need to become adept at dealing with them.

REVIEWING STEP 3

At each review session you should study your monitoring records and ask yourself the following questions in addition to those relating to Steps 1 and 2 (see box below).

1. Have I devised a list of alternative activities? You should have created a list of alternative activities and be carrying it with you. If you are to intervene when you need to, you will need this list at hand. The list may well require amendment on the basis of experience: Some activities may work; others may not.

2. Am I recording urges to eat between my planned meals and snacks? You should have been recording such urges in column 6 of your monitoring records. If you are to intervene suc-

Review Checklist for Step 3

- Have I been monitoring?
- Can I improve my monitoring?
- Are any patterns in my eating becoming obvious?
- Am I weighing myself once a week?
- Each day am I planning regular meals and snacks?
- Am I trying to restrict my eating to the day's meals and snacks?
- Am I skipping any of the meals and snacks?
- Are the gaps between my meals and snacks no longer than three to four hours?
- Am I eating between my meals and snacks?
- Am I getting back on track when things go wrong?
- Am I adjusting the timing of my meals and snacks to accommodate special situations?
- Am I following the advice regarding self-induced vomiting and the misuse of laxatives and diuretics?
- Have I devised a list of alternative activities?
- Am I recording urges to eat between my planned meals and snacks?
- When the opportunity arises, am I using my list of alternative activities?
- Could my use of alternative activities be improved?

cessfully, you must record these urges at the time that you experience them rather than sometime afterward.

Look through the monitoring records that you have completed since starting Step 3 to remind yourself whether you have had urges to eat between your meals and snacks. Did you record them when they occurred? If you have been eating at times other than your planned meals and snacks, this suggests that you have had such urges.

3. When the opportunity arises, am I using my list of alternative activities? When you have the urge to eat between your meals and snacks, have you used your list of alternative activities? Obviously you will benefit only if you practice intervening.

4. Could my use of alternative activities be improved? If you have attempted to intervene, how did it go? Did you intervene early enough? Did you engage in one or more of the activities on your list? Which activities worked, and which did not? Have you modified your list accordingly?

Remember also to complete your summary sheet each week. Classify as a "good day" any day on which you monitored accurately, as described in Step 1; you did your best to stick to your planned pattern of eating, as described in Step 2, whether or not you also binged; and you used your list of alternative activities to deal with any urges to eat.

WHEN TO MOVE ON

It is impossible to specify how long you should spend on this step since you may or may not be having opportunities to practice using alternative activities. Certainly, if your review indicates that you are having urges to eat outside your planned meals and snacks, but you are not successfully intervening, you should delay moving on. As stressed already, the successful use of alternative activities requires practice. It is important that you take every opportunity to do so.

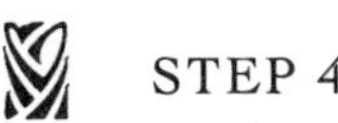 STEP 4

Problem Solving and Taking Stock

BINGES DO NOT GENERALLY OCCUR at random. As described in Chapter 1, they are often triggered by unpleasant events or circumstances. People who binge tend to be particularly prone to do so at times of stress. Therefore, it is important that you develop skills for dealing with those day-to-day problems that might otherwise trigger binges. This is the goal of Step 4.

Do you binge in response to problems? To answer this question you need to review your monitoring records and consider the circumstances surrounding your binges. If you can see that binges tend to be triggered by outside events, you need to develop your problem solving skills. Even if your binges are not generally triggered by external forces, most people find that problem solving skills are useful in many areas, so working on them can only enhance your life.

PROBLEM SOLVING

How to Solve Problems

Efficient problem solving requires six steps:

Step 1—Identify the problem as early as possible. Spotting problems early prevents them from overwhelming you. In the example used in Step 3 (pp. 172–3), you should have spotted the problem—having nothing planned for the evening—during the afternoon, when you were looking ahead. Next best would be spotting the problem as soon as it occurred, say on finishing your evening meal.

The Six Steps of Efficient Problem Solving

Step 1. Identify the problem as early as possible.
Step 2. Specify the problem accurately.
Step 3. Consider as many solutions as possible.
Step 4. Think through the implications of each solution.
Step 5. Choose the best solution or combination of solutions.
Step 6. Act on the solution.

Afterward, review the entire problem solving process.

You may receive clues that a problem is developing. Maybe you are feeling fed up or beginning to have an urge to binge. *Urges to binge are usually a sure sign that there is a problem,* so whenever you have such an urge you should look for the problem behind it.

Sometimes you will find that there is more than one problem. When this is the case, separate the two and deal with them independently, since their solutions may differ.

Step 2—Specify the problem accurately. Working out the true nature of a problem is essential if you are to find the right solution. In the preceding example (pp. 172–3), you might feel that the problem is the fact that you have an urge to binge. Actually that urge is your reaction to the true problem, which is that you have nothing to do all evening and you are tired. So the problem is "I have nothing to do this evening and I am tired."

Step 3—Consider as many solutions as possible. Do not censor yourself at this stage; try to think of all possible solutions. You are more likely to come up with a good one if you do so. Returning to our example, you might come up with these potential solutions:

- Watch TV
- Go to bed
- Go for a jog
- Call some friends to see if they are free
- Clean the apartment
- Go for a drive

Step 4—Think through the implications of each solution. Staying with our example, here are the potential ramifications of adopting each solution listed:

- Watch TV—This is not a great idea since there is nothing worth watching and I will therefore get bored. This will make the risk of binge eating even greater.

- Go to bed—This is also not a good idea. It is how I react when I am fed up, but it solves nothing. Indeed, it makes me feel worse. What tends to happen is that it makes me feel even sorrier for myself. It makes me feel like a failure, and eventually I get up and binge.
- Go for a jog—This is not a bad idea in principle, but given my present weight I don't enjoy jogging. I feel uncomfortable, and I look awful. I suppose that instead I could go for a brisk walk. This would serve the same function since it would help me let off steam while I would also feel good about having exercised.
- Call some friends to see if they are free—This is not a bad idea either. When I feel this way, I usually hide away, but if someone calls me it often cheers me up, especially if we can arrange to meet. Why should I wait for them to call me? I could just as well call them. If they are busy, they can always say so.
- Clean the apartment—The apartment certainly does need cleaning, but I am tired and it is the end of the day. I don't have to do "productive" things all the time.
- Go for a drive—This would be risky. Driving aimlessly around would be bound to end up with my buying food and eating it. This is not a good idea.

Step 5—Choose the best solution or combination of solutions. Choosing the best solution is often not difficult. If you have come up with a number of potential solutions and carefully thought through their implications, the best solution or combination of solutions is usually obvious.

Returning to the example, you decide that calling some friends and then exercising are the best solutions. Note that they are the alternative activities that were chosen in our example in Step 3 of the program. When this happens, they are likely to be particularly effective.

Step 6—Act on the solution. The final step is to act. You do not have to stick rigidly to the chosen solution, however. If it turns out not to be a good idea, the solutions that you considered at Steps 3 and 4 of the problem solving process should have given you other options

Looking back. To become an efficient problem solver, you must take one crucial final step: ***Review the entire problem solving process afterward, usually the next day, to see whether you could have done it any better.*** It is important to stress that the issue is not whether you solved the individual problem, although this is relevant, but rather whether your problem solving could have been any better. Maybe you overcame the problem but didn't problem-solve very well (for example, you thought of just one possible solution and got on with it). While this might feel like a success, it is a short-term way of looking at things. It is important to remember that *the goal is to become good at problem solving in general so that you have this skill at hand for dealing with future difficulties.*

Returning to our example, say you first called three friends, one of whom you had not spoken to for some time. Two of them were in. Neither was free to meet there and then, but you caught up with each other's news and made arrangements to meet in the next week or so. You then forced yourself to go out for a long fast walk. You were out for nearly forty-five minutes. This made you feel tired, but in a different way from how you had been feeling before. You felt healthier and happier, and the urge to binge had gone. You then had a long shower. By this time it was 9:15 P.M. and time for your planned evening snack. After the snack you decided to watch TV for an hour even if there was nothing worth watching and then have an early night. This you did.

The next day you reviewed your problem solving. You considered each step one by one. You thought that you could have done better at identifying the problem as early as possible. Looking back, you saw that it would have been perfectly possible to spot the problem in the afternoon, before you left work. On the other hand, you dealt with the other five steps pretty well. It certainly demonstrated that you could intervene in such a situation, whereas previously you simply would have had a binge and then felt even worse.

What You Should Do

Practice problem solving. From now on, watch out for problems, and each time you identify one, work through the six steps and then review the entire process the following day.

It is a good idea to use your monitoring records to help you solve problems. Write "problem" in column 6 and then turn the sheet of paper over and write out the six steps on the back. Also write out the findings of your review the following day. Figures 21 and 22 show monitoring records that illustrate the example discussed.

REVIEWING STEP 4

At each review session from now on, you should also assess your progress at problem solving. Ask yourself the following questions in addition to those from Steps 1–3 (see box on p. 185).

1. Am I problem solving frequently enough? It is important to look for all opportunities to use your problem solving skills, whether or not the problem might lead to a binge. Any problem, however trivial, will provide you with a chance to develop these skills.

You might feel that problem solving is tedious or pedantic and not your style. Nevertheless, it is worth the effort and will not have to be continued forever. Many people are surprised at how useful they find the technique. Some continue with it long after their eating problems have gone. On the other hand, others abandon it once it no longer seems relevant. For now, it is important that you practice problem solving.

2. When I am problem solving, am I doing it properly? It is important that you follow the six steps. I strongly recommend writing down each step on the back of your monitoring record since doing so will help you think more clearly and will also assist the review process afterward.

3. Am I reviewing my problem solving the next day? Re-

Breakfast – 8:00
Lunch – 12:30
Aft. snack – 3:00
Dinner – 6:30
Eve snack – 9:00

Day . . Monday . . . . Date . . November 3 . . . .

Time	Food and drink consumed	Place	*	V/L	Context and comments
8:30	Coffee Bowl granola	Kitchen			
10:45	Coffee	Work			Very busy at work. Too much to do. Will have to take a short lunch.
12:40	Soup – tomato, slice brown bread, orange Coffee	Cafe			
3:15	1 KitKat	Work			Tired. Too much stress.
6:45	Lasagne – large helping Salad, New potatoes				Left over from yesterday. Eaten too much. I'm tired and there's a long evening ahead of me. Strong urge to binge. PROBLEM → Plan Call friends exercise
9:15	Bowl fruit salad				Left over from yesterday. Early night.

Figure 21. A monitoring record showing a "problem."

1. —

2. I have nothing to do all evening and I'm tired.

3. - TV
 - go to bed
 - jog
 - call friends
 - clean apartment
 - go for drive

4. TV – nothing worth watching, risky
 bed – will make me feel worse
 jog – too hard; could walk instead; nice evening; will let off steam
 call friends – good idea; I ought to do this
 clean apartment – not the right time; the day's been bad enough already!
 drive – pointless and risky

5. Call friends, then exercise

Review: Could have spotted problem earlier – at 3:15 pm. Otherwise did well for first time. Avoided a certain binge. Walking is a good idea – must do it more often.

Figure 22. The back of a monitoring record showing a successful attempt at problem solving.

Review Checklist for Step 4

- Have I been monitoring?
- Can I improve my monitoring?
- Are any patterns in my eating becoming obvious?
- Am I weighing myself once a week?
- Each day am I planning regular meals and snacks?
- Am I trying to restrict my eating to the day's meals and snacks?
- Am I skipping any of the meals and snacks?
- Are the gaps between my meals and snacks no longer than three to four hours?
- Am I eating between my meals and snacks?
- Am I getting back on track when things go wrong?
- Am I adjusting the timing of my meals and snacks to accommodate special situations?
- Am I following the advice regarding self-induced vomiting and the misuse of laxatives and diuretics?
- Have I devised a list of alternative activities?
- Am I recording urges to eat between my planned meals and snacks?
- When the opportunity arises, am I using my list of alternative activities?
- Could my use of alternative activities be improved?
- Am I problem solving frequently enough?
- When I problem-solve, am I doing it properly?
- Am I reviewing my problem solving the next day?

viewing each attempt at problem solving is central to developing your problem solving skills. It is important to remember that the issue is not whether the individual problem was solved (although hopefully it was) but rather whether you followed the six steps as well as you could. Could your problem solving have been any better?

Remember also to continue to complete your summary sheet each week. You will need this for taking stock, the next part of Step 4.

Classify as a "good day" any day on which you monitored accurately, as described in Step 1; you did your best to stick to your planned pattern of eating, as described in Step 2, whether or not you also binged; you used your list of alternative activities to deal with any urges to eat, as described in Step 3; and you practiced problem solving at every available opportunity, as described here.

WHEN TO MOVE ON

As before, it is not possible to provide specific guidelines for when to move on since you may or may not be having opportunities to develop your problem solving skills. Remember, though, that any problem can be used for practicing, not just those that are liable to trigger binges.

TAKING STOCK

This is the point in the program when you should stand back and review your progress in detail. To do so you will need your summary sheet.

Is the Program Helping?

By now, if the program is going to help you, you should see definite signs that you are benefiting. Three main outcomes are likely. Work out which applies to you.

Outcome 1. If the frequency of your binges has clearly decreased (and, if applicable, so has your vomiting and/or use of laxatives or diuretics), you should continue with the program. These are very promising signs, and you are doing well.

Outcome 2. If you are doing your best to change, a good measure of which is the number of good days you are having each week, yet the frequency of your binges has not changed significantly, the program is not right for you. Instead, you should seriously consider getting outside help.

Outcome 3. If you are not benefiting in terms of your eating, but you can also see that you are not following the program as well as you could, you need to question your commitment to change. It would be a good idea to reread the section "Why Change?" at the beginning of Part II. If you decide that you really do want to change, you should seriously consider restarting the program, perhaps after a short break. On the other hand, if you are unsure whether you want to change—perhaps it all seems to take too much effort or this is the wrong time—it might be better to stop for the meantime. You can always restart at some point in the future.

Changes in Weight

By now it should also be clear what is happening to your weight. Most people find that there has been little or no change, although there may have been fluctuations from week to week.

If your weight has decreased by more than five pounds, it is important to check that you are not now underweight (see Table 8 in the Introduction to Part II). If you are, see your physician, explain what you have been doing, and get advice. You must consider whether you are losing weight because you are eating too little in your meals and snacks. This is a potential problem since it will limit your progress. This issue is dealt with in detail in Step 5.

If your weight has increased by more than about five pounds, you need to check two things. The first is whether the weight gain is arising because you are recovering from having been underweight. You may have started the program at a low weight compared to your natural weight, and now that you are beginning to eat more healthily your weight is returning to its natural level. This is a good thing although you may be finding it difficult to tolerate. Remember that at this stage *it is best if you concentrate your efforts on overcoming the binge eating problem and accept whatever changes in weight occur.* As discussed earlier, if you do this, your weight will gradually move toward its natural level, which may be lower than, higher than, or much the same as its current level. And this is the weight that you should do your best to accept since fighting it will mean an endless battle against your biology, a battle you will never win.

The second point to check if your weight has increased is whether you are now "overweight," medically speaking. Appendix II explains how to tell and provides specific advice if this is the case.

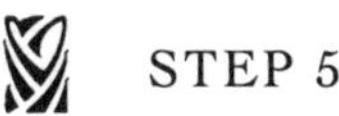

STEP 5

Dieting and Related Forms of Food Avoidance

By now your binge eating problem should be showing definite signs of improvement. Introducing the pattern of regular eating (Step 2) should have had the effect of displacing binges, and resisting urges to binge by engaging in alternative activities (Step 3) should have further reduced their frequency. Problem solving (Step 4) should be helping you stop binge eating in response to day-to-day difficulties.

To build on your progress and maintain it, you need to tackle any general vulnerability to binge. If your binges are triggered primarily by stress, problem solving in combination with eating at regular intervals and using alternative activities will often be sufficient. On the other hand, it is dieting that makes many people prone to binge.

Chapter 4 described three forms of dieting: avoiding eating for long periods of time, restricting the overall amount of food eaten, and avoiding eating certain types of food. All three are common among those who binge, and all three tend to encourage binge eating. This is particularly true if the dieting is *strict*—governed by highly specific rules that tend to be applied in an all-or-nothing fashion. Strict dieters tend to impose on themselves a variety of demanding dietary rules, and they respond to the breaking of these rules by giving up and overeating. As a result they alternate between dieting and binge eating with each encouraging the other.

To determine whether you are a strict dieter, review your monitoring records to get answers to the following two groups of questions:

1. What do you eat outside your binges? Are you purposely restricting what you eat? If so, what is the nature of your diet? Are you attempting to follow any particular regimen? For example, are you trying not to eat for long periods of time? Are you attempting to limit the overall amount you eat, perhaps by staying below a set calorie limit? Are you avoiding particular types of food, ones that you view as fattening? And, most important, are you diet-

ing in an all-or-nothing way, such that if you break your diet you give up and binge?

2. What triggers your binges? Are they triggered by your failing to follow personal dietary rules? For example, do they occur if you eat more than you feel you ought to? Are they triggered by eating banned or forbidden foods?

If your answer to these questions is yes, it is essential that you stop dieting in this way. Otherwise you will remain prone to binge.

HOW TO DEAL WITH STRICT DIETING

The three types of dieting call for three different approaches to stopping.

Trying Not to Eat for Long Periods of Time

You've already taken measures to tackle this behavior by establishing a pattern of regular eating at Step 2. If you used to try not to eat for long periods of time, it is essential that you start to eat at regular intervals through the day. On the other hand, it is important that you remain flexible. The recommended pattern of eating is not meant to be rigid; it provides only general guidelines.

Trying to Restrict the Overall Amount of Food You Eat

The tendency to limit how much you eat—such as by setting a calorie limit—must be countered for two reasons. First, such dietary restriction is often so extreme that it inevitably encourages binge eating as a result of physiological pressures to eat. Certainly any diet that involves eating 1,200 calories a day or less will have this effect. Second, strict dieters set themselves very specific dietary goals, and they are prone to binge if they do not meet them.

So, eating anything at all over 1,200 calories will represent failure to someone who is trying to keep to a 1,200-calorie diet.

To tackle this form of dieting, you must first decide whether there is any need for you to restrict your calorie intake. *There is no need for most people with binge eating problems to diet;* indeed, it is unwise for them to do so since dieting makes them vulnerable to binge. (See Appendix II if you binge and are overweight.) Assuming that there is no good reason for you to diet, you should try to stop dieting. You should stop attempting to restrict the overall amount that you eat and, if applicable, stop counting calories. Paradoxically, this may well result in your eating less, since you will be less prone to binge.

If you are afraid that you will overeat if you stop dieting, then you may need guidelines to determine what is a "normal" amount to eat. As mentioned in Step 2, you could identify people of about your age (and gender) and see what they eat or you could follow the advice on food packages and in recipes. (A friend or relative who is helping you with the program could also advise you.)

Trying to Avoid Certain Types of Food

It is especially important to tackle this form of dieting since it is particularly likely to lead people to binge. Avoiding foods—and often there are a great many of them—results in a narrowly restricted diet, and it makes people feel deprived. And, of course, eating these foods is one of the major triggers of binges.

In principle, food avoidance is the easiest form of dieting to tackle since all you have to do is introduce these foods into your diet. In practice, however, this is often easier said than done. For example, you may have become so used to not eating certain foods that you are no longer aware you are avoiding them. A first step therefore is to identify any foods you are denying yourself. The best way of doing this may seem rather odd, but it works. Go to a local supermarket that stocks most types and brands of food, and walk up and down the aisles, writing down in a notebook (other shoppers will think you are an employee!) all the foods (that you like) that you would be reluctant to eat, either because of the effect they might have on your weight or shape or because you think eating them might trigger a binge. Then, at home, organize this list of foods (often it contains 40 or more items) into three or four groups according to the degree of difficulty that you would have eating them.

The next step is gradually to introduce these foods into your diet. Do so by including them in your planned meals and snacks. Do this only on days on which you feel in control, since otherwise they might trigger a binge. Start by introducing foods from the easiest of your three or four groups and focus on them for a couple of weeks. Then move to the next group and so on. Within six to eight weeks you should have incorporated all the foods into your diet. It usually does not matter how much of the food that you eat. Even a little will do. It tends to be the idea of having eaten the food that triggers binges rather than the amount itself.

Some people find doing this easy, but others do not. Either way, it requires sustained practice. You should keep introducing these foods until you no longer find it difficult. *The time when you can stop is when eating these avoided foods no longer unsettles you. If you are not avoiding any foods, you are much less likely to binge.*

Of course, following this advice involves your eating foods that you may regard as fattening or unhealthy. It is important that you persevere nonetheless. No foods are inherently fattening; it all depends on the amount of them that you eat. Introducing these foods will enhance your control over eating since you will be less likely to binge. As to their unhealthiness, it is clearly preferable to eat such foods in moderation than to eat large quantities in an uncontrolled fashion.

A point worth stressing is that you will not need to eat these foods forever. Rather, as soon as doing so stops making you anxious it would be reasonable to cut back on those foods that are accepted to be unhealthy (fats and simple carbohydrates—see Appendix II and Further Reading), although it would be best not to exclude them altogether. In the long term you should be able to allow yourself to eat anything at times—nothing should be rigidly banned.

HOW TO DEAL WITH RELATED FORMS OF AVOIDANCE

Most forms of dieting are, in essence, avoiding eating to influence appearance or weight. But many people with binge eating problems avoid other situations related to eating, and this may also perpetuate binge eating problems. Two common examples are avoiding eating with other people and avoiding eating foods when you're uncertain of their calorie content.

To overcome your binge eating problem, it is important that you tackle all forms of avoidance of eating. It should be obvious what situations you are avoiding. You just have to ask yourself whether there are any situations involving eating that make you anxious. If so, you need to address them.The way to tackle such anxiety-provoking situations is the same in principle as that for tackling food avoidance. You work out a graded plan for introducing yourself to these situations in a way that will not cause you undue stress. For example, to tackle anxiety over eating with others, you might establish the following progressive goals:

1. Eat at home with the friend/relative who is helping you with the program.
2. Eat in an unthreatening restaurant with this person.
3. Eat in an unthreatening restaurant with another person with whom you are comfortable.
4. Eat in an unthreatening restaurant with people who are prone to make you anxious (e.g., your parents).
5. Eat in a threatening environment with people who are prone to make you anxious (e.g., eat at home with your parents).

Then start at the easiest (or least difficult) level and practice it. Once you can accomplish it without undue anxiety, you should move on to the next level and practice it, and so on. You have finished the process once you have practiced so often that the overall situation no longer makes you particularly anxious and you no longer wish to avoid it.

What You Should Do

Unless you do not diet, start following the guidelines for dealing with the three forms of dieting. Assess your progress at each review session. Remember to consider each of the forms of dieting. In addition, if you are avoiding other situations involving eating, you should set up a hierarchy as described above and systematically work your way through it.

REVIEWING STEP 5

At each of your review sessions, inspect your monitoring records to assess your progress at tackling dieting and related forms of avoidance. Ask yourself the following two questions in addition to the questions relating to the previous steps in the program (see box on p. 196):

1. ***Am I tackling the three forms of dieting?***
   - Trying not to eat for long periods of time
   - Trying to restrict the overall amount eaten
   - Trying to avoid certain types of food

2. ***Am I tackling other forms of avoidance?*** If the answer is no to any of these questions, reread the guidelines in Step 5.

You should also continue to complete your summary sheet each week. Classify as a "good day" any day on which you monitored accurately, as described in Step 1; you did your best to stick to your planned pattern of eating, as described in Step 2, whether or not you also binged; you used your list of alternative activities to deal with any urges to eat, as described in Step 3; you practiced

Review Checklist for Step 5

- Have I been monitoring?
- Can I improve my monitoring?
- Are any patterns in my eating becoming obvious?
- Am I weighing myself once a week?
- Each day am I planning regular meals and snacks?
- Am I trying to restrict my eating to the day's meals and snacks?
- Am I skipping any of the meals and snacks?
- Are the gaps between my meals and snacks no longer than three to four hours?
- Am I eating between my meals and snacks?
- Am I getting back on track when things go wrong?
- Am I adjusting the timing of my meals and snacks to accommodate special situations?
- Am I following the advice regarding self-induced vomiting and the misuse of laxatives and diuretics?
- Have I devised a list of alternative activities?
- Am I recording urges to eat between my planned meals and snacks?
- When the opportunity arises, am I using my list of alternative activities?
- Could my use of alternative activities be improved?
- Am I problem solving frequently enough?
- When I problem solve, am I doing it properly?
- Am I reviewing my problem solving the next day?
- Am I eating at regular intervals through the day?
- Am I eating normal quantities of food, or am I restricting the overall amount that I eat?
- Am I able to eat any food (that I like) without feeling anxious?
- Am I tackling other forms of avoidance?

problem solving at every available opportunity, as described in Step 4; and you tackled any remaining tendency to diet, as described here.

WHEN TO MOVE ON

It usually takes some time to get out of the habit of dieting, at least a month or two and often longer. There is no rush. On the other hand, do push yourself. ***Until you stop dieting, you will remain vulnerable to bingeing.*** And it may take several additional weeks or months to deal with related forms of avoidance.

Once you have completed these tasks, you are nearing the end of the program. It is therefore time to take stock once again. To do so, move on to Step 6.

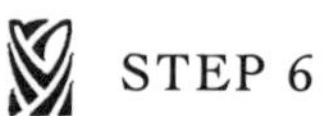

What Next?

Step 1: Getting Started
Self-monitoring
Weekly weighing

Step 2: Regular Eating
Establishing a pattern of regular eating
Stopping vomiting and misusing laxatives and diuretics

Step 3: Alternatives to Binge Eating
Substituting alternative activities

Step 4: Problem Solving and Taking Stock
Practicing problem solving
Reviewing progress

Step 5: Dieting and Related Forms of Avoidance
Tackling the three forms of dieting
Tackling other forms of avoidance of eating

Step 6: What Next?
Preventing relapse
Dealing with other problems

NOW THAT YOU HAVE NEARLY completed the program, it is time to take stock once again. What you should do next depends on the degree to which you have benefited. When taking stock, it is best to separate your binge eating problem from other ongoing difficulties. It is also important to appreciate that matters will not necessarily remain static. While I will be focusing on preventing relapse in describing Step 6, you should understand that the more common state of affairs is continuing improvement. This is because the program disrupts the vicious circles that keep the binge eating problem going, and the fruits of this process sometimes take many months to be fully expressed.

THE BINGE EATING PROBLEM

If Binge Eating Is Still a Problem

If binge eating is still interfering with your quality of life, you should seriously consider getting further help. The options were described at the beginning of Part II of this book. The fact that the self-help program did not help or did so only to a limited degree, does not mean that the problem cannot be overcome. Far from it. There are many other treatment options, and you must not give up.

If You Have Improved or Recovered

In the short term—for about the next six months—you should continue to employ the strategies that you have found most helpful. Also continue to hold regular review sessions, perhaps every two weeks, to assess your progress.

It is impossible to give firm recommendations regarding when to stop monitoring your eating. The best advice is to stop when it is no longer relevant. However, you must beware of stopping because you do not want to face up to the fact that you still have problems or that things are deteriorating. On the other hand, if your eating is stable and satisfactory, there is no need to monitor.

Taking a longer-term perspective, the key issue is how to ensure that you will maintain and build on the changes you have made. There are four aspects to this process:

1. Having realistic expectations
2. Distinguishing a lapse from a relapse
3. Knowing how to deal with setbacks
4. Reducing vulnerability

PREVENTING RELAPSE

Having Realistic Expectations

It is common for people who have stopped binge eating to hope that they will never binge again. While this hope is understandable, it is neither helpful nor realistic. You should regard your eating problem as an Achilles' heel. You will still be prone to react this way at times of stress. With luck it will be very much in the background and will not affect your everyday life. Nevertheless, it may recur, and you need to be prepared.

Also common among people who have stopped binge eating is the view that they should start dieting to lose weight now that they have control over their eating. As explained earlier, however, strict dieting puts people at risk of bingeing, the return of which will run counter to any weight loss efforts. If you are truly overweight, Appendix II describes various realistic options for losing weight. Remember, though, that for the great majority of people it is better to learn to live with your weight than to risk an endless battle with your biology—a battle you can never win.

Distinguishing a Lapse from a Relapse

How you deal with future problems is central to the successful prevention of relapses. A particularly important distinction to be made is that between a lapse and a relapse. A lapse is a setback or slip, whereas a relapse is returning to square one. The two terms have different connotations. Implicit in the notion of a lapse is the idea that there can be degrees of deterioration. On the other hand the notion of a relapse suggests that one has either recovered or not. This type of thinking should be familiar by now; it is another example of all-or-nothing (dichotomous) thinking, a thinking style that is common among those who binge.

To minimize the chances of relapsing, it is important not to label lapses as relapses, since doing so is likely to affect your behavior. If you think you have had a lapse, you are likely to take steps to get back on track. If you regard yourself as having relapsed, you may well give up, and as a result matters will get worse.

Knowing How to Deal with Setbacks

1. Spot the problem early. It should be obvious if things are deteriorating since the frequency of your binge eating will increase. Your task, therefore, is to respond to any such increase. Do not turn a blind eye, hoping that the setback will be temporary. Instead, assume that there is a problem and take steps to do something about it.

2. Reinstitute the program. To nip the lapse in the bud, it is important that you reinstitute the program as soon as possible. Be your own therapist. Reread the program and restart monitoring and whatever other procedures seem appropriate. Review your progress every few days. Problems caught early are much easier to solve than those that have been allowed to take hold.

3. Identify any source of stress. It may be obvious what has led to the setback, or it may not be at all clear. Either way, think carefully about what might have precipitated the problem and tackle it using the problem solving approach described in Step 4 of the program. Again, review your progress every few days.

With this three-pronged approach, you can overcome most lapses. If you are not succeeding, however, do not delay seeking professional help.

Reducing Vulnerability

While it is impossible to protect yourself from all external stresses, you can reduce the risk that you will respond by binge eating.

You can do this by making sure that you are not dieting since dieting makes people vulnerable to binge. ***To minimize the chances that your binge eating problem will return, do your best not to resume dieting.***

DEALING WITH OTHER PROBLEMS

As described in Chapter 4, most binge eating problems do not exist in isolation. Rather, they are accompanied by a range of other difficulties, such as concerns about appearance and weight, feelings of depression and anxiety, and problems with relationships. As also explained, it is usual for such associated problems to improve substantially, if not resolve altogether, as the binge eating problem improves. But this does not always happen.

It is beyond the scope of this book to provide a detailed account of ways to deal with such problems, but the following suggestions should help.

Excessive Concern about Appearance or Weight

Many people today are concerned about their appearance or weight or both. Most would like to look thinner and weigh less. For some this is an overriding concern that dominates their life and is clearly excessive. It is above and beyond the "normal" level of dissatisfaction discussed in Chapter 4. Extreme concerns of this type are not unusual among those with binge eating problems, and by definition they are always present in those with anorexia nervosa or bulimia nervosa.

Concerns about appearance and weight tend to be magnified and maintained by binge eating problems. It is hardly surprising that repeated episodes of uncontrolled eating (binges) intensify fears of fatness and weight gain. And these fears encourage dieting, which in turn encourages binge eating, and so a vicious circle operates.

If this program has been of help, you will have experienced a significant decrease in your frequency of binge eating. This in turn may well have resulted in a lessening of your concerns about appearance and weight, in part because your control over eating will have improved and in part because your morale and self-confidence will have been enhanced. In some cases, however, such concerns remain a problem. If this applies, what should you do?

It is important that you try to tackle these concerns. Not doing so endangers the progress that you have made, because it is difficult to stop dieting when you are still afraid of weight gain or fatness. Two books can help you address these concerns: *Making Peace with Food* by Susan Kano is a self-help book for those with eating problems. It focuses in particular on improving attitudes toward shape and weight and enhancing self-acceptance. *Body Traps* by Judith Rodin provides a clear and up-to-date account of what is known about such concerns as well as exercises for dealing with them. If you are a woman, in addition to this book, you may find it helpful to read some feminist writing on the subject. *The Beauty Myth* by Naomi Wolf is especially good. Two other well-known books are *Fat Is a Feminist Issue* by Susie Orbach and *The Hungry Self* by Kim Chernin. A book that may be of special interest to women who are overweight is *Being Fat Is Not a Sin* by Shelley Bovey. (Details on all of these books are in Further Reading.)

If your concerns about appearance and weight persist and are severe despite your attempts to moderate them, you should seek specialized help. (See "How to Change: The Various Options" at the beginning of Part II.)

Problems with Depression, Anxiety, and Low Self-Esteem

As explained in Chapter 4, problems with depression, anxiety, and low self-esteem usually improve as binge eating problems improve. However, this does not always happen. If you still have such problems, and they are interfering significantly with your day-to-day life, you should seek professional help. If they are not quite so severe, two books by David Burns may prove helpful. *Feeling Good* focuses on depression and low self-esteem, but it also has a useful section on perfectionism. *The Feeling Good Handbook* addresses depression and low self-esteem but in addition deals with anxiety and relationship problems. A book that is good on various forms of negative thinking is *When Am I Going to Be Happy* by Penelope Russianoff.

Relationship Problems

Difficulties with relationships are also not uncommon among those with binge eating problems. They have a variety of causes. Some may have preceded the eating problem and have contributed to it, whereas others may have arisen since the problem developed and be, at least in part, the result of it.

When binge eating problems improve, the effect on relationships varies. Some improve, some remain unchanged, and some even worsen. If you have significant relationship problems and a central issue is faulty communication, then *The Feeling Good Handbook* may help. Problems with assertiveness are addressed in *When I Say No, I Feel Guilty* by Manuel Smith, and problems with shyness and loneliness are the focus of another book by David Burns titled *Intimate Connections*.

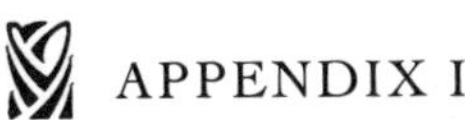

APPENDIX I

The Body Mass Index

THANKS TO THE BELGIAN astronomer Quetelet, there is a simple means for determining whether someone is underweight, a healthy weight, or overweight. This is to calculate the person's so-called body mass index or BMI. The resulting figure will be between 10 and 50. Here is how to interpret it:

Under 16: extremely underweight
16–18: significantly underweight
20–25: healthy weight
27–30: overweight
30–40: significantly overweight
Over 40: extremely overweight

The ranges 18 to 20 and 25 to 27 are gray areas that represent being slightly underweight and slightly overweight respectively. *All these thresholds apply to both men and women (over the age of 16 years) whatever their build.*

APPENDIX I

HOW TO CALCULATE YOUR OWN BMI

Calculating your own BMI is simple, but you will need a calculator.

1. Multiply your weight (in pounds) by 700.
2. Divide the answer by your height (in inches).
3. Once more divide the answer by your height (in inches). The resulting figure is your BMI.*

Here is an example. Say you are 5 feet 4 inches tall (64 inches) and weigh 120 pounds:

1. 120 × 700 = 84,000
2. 84,000 ÷ 64 = 1,312.5
3. 1,312.5 ÷ 64 = 20.5

Your BMI is therefore 20.5 (i.e., your weight is in the healthy range).

From the perspective of this book, two BMIs are of particular significance: 18 (the threshold for being underweight) and 27 (the threshold for being overweight). To simplify matters, Tables 8 (see Introduction to Part II) and 9 (see Appendix II) list the weights for various heights that are equivalent to these two BMIs.

---

*The three steps are equivalent to the following calculation:

$$\text{BMI} = \frac{\text{Weight (in kilograms)}}{\text{Height (in meters) x Height (in meters)}}$$

APPENDIX II

If You Are Overweight

MANY PEOPLE WITH BINGE EATING problems are overweight. While the relationship between binge eating and obesity is complex and ill understood (see Chapter 5), it is clear that the two problems interact and exacerbate each other (see Chapter 6). Binge eating is likely to contribute to the maintenance of obesity, and it certainly makes treatment more difficult. Conversely, those treatments for obesity that involve strict dieting can have a tendency to make binge eating problems worse.

Body weight is not as easy to control as is generally thought. It is strongly determined by genetic factors. It is therefore not surprising that dieting and behavioral treatments for obesity have little effect in the long term. (For a careful analysis of the effectiveness of these methods, see the article by Dr G. Terence Wilson of Rutgers University listed in Further Reading.) The claims of the diet industry are now coming under public scrutiny, and many are being shown to be exaggerated. Where does this leave people who are overweight?

To answer this question, it is important to define *overweight*. While the dictates of current fashion would class most women as overweight, health risks reach significance only at a body mass index above 27. (Appendix I explains the body mass index and how to calculate your own.) Table 9 shows what weights in pounds are equivalent to a body mass index of 27 (for different heights). If you weigh more than the weight shown for your height, you are "overweight" in medical terms. As a consequence, you are at increased risk of a range of health problems including high blood pressure, heart disease, and diabetes. If your body mass index is over 30, your risk of these problems is markedly increased. On the other hand, if your body mass index is below 27, you are not

Table 9. Are You Overweight?

Below is a list of weights for various different heights. These represent a body mass index of 27 (see Appendix I for an explanation). They apply to men and women. To determine whether you are overweight, find your height on the table and look across at the weight for that height. If you weigh more than this weight, your body mass index is over 27 and you are medically overweight.

Height[a] (feet, inches)	Weight[b] (pounds)	Height[a] (feet, inches)	Weight[b] (pounds)
4'10"	128	5'8"	178
4'10½"	132	5'8½"	179
4'11"	134	5'9"	182
4'11½"	135	5'9½"	186
5'0"	137	5'10"	188
5'½"	139	5'10½"	190
5'1"	143	5'11"	192
5'1½"	144	5'11½"	197
5'2"	148	6'0"	198
5'2½"	150	6'½"	201
5'3"	152	6'1"	203
5'3½"	154	6'1½"	207
5'4"	157	6'2"	210
5'4½"	159	6'2½"	212
5'5"	162	6'3"	216
5'5½"	163	6'3½"	219
5'6"	168	6'4"	221
5'6½"	169	6'4½"	223
5'7"	172	6'5"	228
5'7½"	175	6'5½"	230

[a]Without shoes.
[b]Without shoes, light indoor clothing.

overweight medically speaking. Nevertheless, you may want to lose some weight for other reasons.

If you are medically overweight as defined here, it is entirely appropriate that you take note of the associated health risks and try to minimize them. There are several things you can do. One is to ensure that you are reasonably fit. Another is to follow a healthy diet. Neither of these tasks requires you to lose weight (although weight loss may occur), yet both can reduce the health risks associated with obesity. You may, of course, also want to lose some weight, for health or other reasons, but if you have a binge eating problem, it is important to think twice before actively trying to do so since, as already mentioned, some weight control treatments make binge eating worse. If you do decide to attempt to lose weight, it is important that you take the following advice.

AN IMPORTANT DECISION— WHICH SHOULD YOU TACKLE FIRST?

If you are overweight and binge eat, you have two problems, an eating problem and a weight problem. Tackling both at once is difficult, so which should you address first?

While your first priority may be to tackle your weight problem, this is not necessarily the best first step. The key issue is whether tackling your weight will worsen your binge eating. If you have adopted weight control programs in the past and found that your progress is undermined by your binge eating, you should tackle the binge eating first. If this is not the case, you could start by tackling your weight problem (following the guidelines here) and see what happens to your binge eating.

TACKLING YOUR BINGE EATING

To tackle your binge eating, *you need to follow the program exactly as specified in Part II of this book.* All the steps apply, although the advice regarding vomiting and the misuse of laxatives and diuretics may not be relevant. The step that you may find most difficult is that aimed at eliminating strict dieting (Step 5). You may have been struggling with your weight for many years, and dieting may seem part of your life. To stop dieting may feel like giving up and abandoning yourself to obesity. This is not the case, however, since your binge eating problem is likely to have been made worse by your attempts to diet, and the binge eating may be contributing to your obesity. So, paradoxically, you may be more likely to lose weight by not dieting than by continually trying to diet.

It is particularly important that you introduce any avoided foods into your diet since food avoidance is especially prone to encourage binge eating. If you have been told that you are "addicted" to certain foods and must therefore permanently avoid them, reread Chapter 7. Contrary to the claims of some groups, there is no scientific evidence that certain foods have addictive or toxic properties.

In addition to following the program, you will need to make two changes:

1. Establish a physically active lifestyle
2. Eat a healthy diet

ESTABLISHING A PHYSICALLY ACTIVE LIFESTYLE

People who are overweight tend to be less physically active than people who are not overweight. This tendency needs to be addressed since great benefits can come from getting more exercise. Not only are the chances of losing weight enhanced, but the health risks associated with obesity are diminished even in the absence of weight loss.

You should therefore try to establish a generally more active lifestyle. This has been called "opportunistic exercising," and it involves looking for opportunities to exercise whenever you can. One good way of doing this is to include more walking in your day-to-day life. Your goal should be to do more walking on a permanent basis. For example, you could start to make a habit of using stairs rather than elevators; you could park a few blocks away from your destination and at the far end of parking lots; and you could get off the bus a few stops early. This advice might seem mundane, but simple measures of this type, if adopted permanently, will have a significant effect on your level of fitness and overall health.

In addition, you should start a program of regular exercise. It is important that this be realistic so that you can keep it up. Whatever type of exercise you choose, and four good options are listed below, you should follow these guidelines:

1. If your physical health might be impaired in any way, see your doctor before starting the exercise program.
2. Make sure that you wear comfortable clothing. There is no reason to wear tight or revealing outfits.
3. If the exercise involves weight bearing, you must have good-quality athletic shoes.
4. Chart your day-to-day progress on your monitoring records and at the end of each week transfer this information to your summary sheet. (You will need to add a column for this purpose.) The goal should be to start exercising three times a week (initially for ten minutes each session), and then increase the session length by five minutes each week until the sessions last at least twenty minutes and preferably somewhat longer. If possible, you should also aim to increase the number of sessions from three to four a week.
5. Do not exercise intensely. If you are unable to carry out a conversation while exercising, you are working too hard.
6. If you are prone to get bored while exercising, you may find various forms of distraction helpful. For example, if practicable, listen to a portable stereo or radio or watch television.

Some good forms of exercise are listed below. Choose the one that you think you will enjoy most.

- *Walking.* This is a good form of exercise, particularly for those who are significantly overweight. It is not overly strenuous and requires no equipment other than good shoes.
- *Swimming.* This is another excellent form of exercise, particularly for those who have problems weight-bearing. Even if you have not swum for years, you will soon find that the skill returns. The main problem is sensitivity about appearance. A comfortable bathing suit is essential.
- *Indoor skiing.* Indoor skiing machines are popular and are not very expensive. At first it can be difficult to get the knack, but thereafter most people have no trouble at all. It is easy to grade the intensity of the exercising.
- *Strength (resistance) training.* Resistance training (e.g., weight training) is also of value and is relatively easy to learn. A simple routine of exercises is best.

EATING A HEALTHY DIET

The second addition to the program involves establishing a healthy diet. The basic principles are simple:

- Decrease the amount of fats and simple carbohydrates.
- Increase the amount of fiber and complex carbohydrates.

These general guidelines may be translated into the following more specific pieces of advice (for more guidance, see the Further Reading section of this book):

1. Fats, oils, and sweets should be consumed in limited quantities. For example, when cooking, use only small amounts of fats and oils. Also, be sparing in your consumption of butter, margarine, mayonnaise, and salad dressings.

2. No more than 30 percent of your total calorie intake should come from fat (i.e., 60 to 70 grams a day).
3. Whenever possible, use skim or low-fat milk and low-fat yogurt and cheese. Ice cream contains a great deal of fat and should be eaten sparingly.
4. Try to eat lean meat and trim the skin from poultry. Limit your intake of nuts since they are also rich in fat.
5. Experiment with vegetables by eating different types and by trying different ways of preparing them. Regularly eat starchy vegetables (e.g., potatoes) and beans.
6. Make fruit part of your daily diet. Experiment with different types.
7. Bread (whole-grain), cereal, pasta, and rice should be a major part of your diet.

On the other hand, it is important on occasion to allow yourself to eat desserts and other less healthy foods: Indeed, it is to be encouraged since rigidly excluding such foods will make you prone to binge. "Binge-proof" eating involves no rules, just general guidelines.

TACKLING YOUR WEIGHT PROBLEM

As explained, tackling your weight problem is not necessarily the best first step even if it is your top priority. If, in the past, following weight control programs has led to a worsening of your binge eating problem, then you should first address your binge eating problem following the preceding guidelines. On the other hand, if you have no evidence that this is the case, or you have already successfully addressed your binge eating problem, then tackling your weight problem is entirely appropriate. This is especially true if you have a general tendency to overeat (see Chapter 4) since moderating the size and frequency of your meals and snacks is likely to have significant benefits. The weight control program I would recommend is the LEARN program devised by Dr. Kelly Brownell of Yale (see Further Reading). It is tried and tested, focuses on healthy eating and exercise habits, and is unlikely to encourage binge eating. On the other hand, it is probably not advisable to follow extreme weight loss programs involving liquid fasts since they may worsen your eating problem.

What should be your weight goal? One of the reasons that the U.S. Federal Trade Commission is looking into the advertising practices of several commercial diet programs is that they promise there will be substantial and sustained weight loss. The research evidence does not support such claims—again the article by Dr G. Terence Wilson is recommended (see Further Reading)—yet millions of people are blaming themselves for not meeting their weight goals rather than realizing that the goals themselves are at fault. For most people they are unrealistic.

Nowadays clinicians and researchers are advocating that people be helped to accept the weight and shape that result once they have established an active lifestyle, a healthy diet, and regular eating habits. Drs. Janet Polivy and Peter Herman of the University of Toronto refer to this as the body's "natural weight." The term used by Dr. Kelly Brownell is a "reasonable weight," one that is realistic to maintain in the long term. What is your natural or reasonable weight? This is difficult to say. It can be discovered only by making the lifestyle changes suggested and seeing what happens.

I accept that it is difficult to moderate your goal weight to one that is higher than that promised by diet programs. It means turning a blind eye to their seductive claims and, in many cases, giving up the hope of ever being truly slim. But doing so will be so much better for your self-respect and self-confidence than yet more years of struggling with dieting and binge eating and the weight cycles that result.

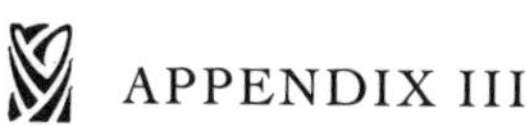

APPENDIX III

Organizations That Can Help

VARIOUS ORGANIZATIONS KEEP a register of professionals who specialize in helping those with eating problems. To find out the names of specialists in your area, contact one of the following organizations. (Many other countries have their own organizations.)

UNITED STATES

National Eating Disorders Organization (NEDO)
445 E. Granville Rd.
Worthington, OH 43085-3195
614-436-1112

National Association of Anorexia Nervosa and Associated Disorders (ANAD)
Box 7
Highland Park, IL 60035
708-831-3438

American Anorexia/Bulimia Association Inc (AABA)
418 E. 76th St.
New York, NY 10021
212-734-1114

Anorexia Nervosa & Related Eating Disorders (ANRED)
PO Box 5102
Eugene, OR 97405
503-344-1144

Another organization of importance is the National Association to Aid Fat Americans, an advocacy and support group that fights all forms of discrimination against fat people.

National Association to Aid Fat Americans (NAAFA)
PO Box 188620
Sacramento, CA 95818
916-443-0303

CANADA

National Eating Disorder Information Centre
200 Elizabeth St.
College Way
Toronto, Ontario M5G 2C4
416-340-4156

Bulimia, Anorexia Nervosa Association (BANA)
3640 Wells St.
Windsor, Ontario N9C 1T9
519-253-7545

UNITED KINGDOM

Eating Disorders Association
Sackville Place
44 Magdalen Street
Norwich
Norfolk NR3 1J3
01603-621414

ITALY

ICED (Italian Centre for Eating Disorders)
Via Ugo Ojetti 16
Flat 4
Rome 00137
6-8689-6825

NORWAY

Anorexia Bulimia Association
pb 36
N-5001 Bergen
5-475167785

SPAIN

ADANER (Asociación en defensa de la atención de la anorexia nervosa)
Calle Mirabel 17, 5 D
28044 Madrid
1-91-5044347 (helpline)

SWITZERLAND

ABA (Association Boulimie–Anorexie)
Ch. des Communailles
CH-1055 Froideville
21-881-30-74

AUSTRALIA

ABNA Inc. (Anorexia Bulimia Nervosa Association, Inc.)
35 Fullarton Rd.
Kent Town
South Australia 5067
8-362-6772

Anorexia and Bulimia Nervosa Foundation of Victoria, Inc.
1513 High St.
Glen Iris 3146
Victoria
613-885-0318

NEW ZEALAND

Eating Difficulties Education Network
PO Box 38-233
Howick
Auckland
9-535-9619

Women with Eating Disorders Resource Centre
PO Box 4520
Armagh and Montreal St.
Christchurch
3-643-366-7725

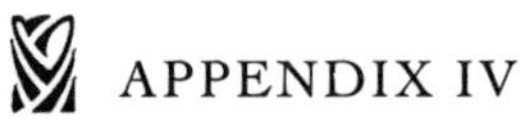

A Note for Relatives and Friends

THIS BOOK PROVIDES AN ACCOUNT of what is known about binge eating problems and their treatment (Part I). It includes a detailed step-by-step self-help program based on the most effective treatment available (Part II).

If you have bought this book because you are concerned that a relative or friend might have a binge eating problem, then the main descriptive chapters (Chapters 1 and 4) should clarify matters. And if you are concerned about the physical effects of binge eating problems, read Chapter 5. Treatment is discussed in Chapter 8.

Perhaps you think your relative or friend has a binge eating problem, but the issue has never been discussed. This is a difficult situation since it is obviously the other person's right to decide whether he or she wishes to talk about the problem and whether he or she wishes to do something about it. Nevertheless, it does seem reasonable to ensure that someone you are concerned about is well informed. An appropriate initial measure would be to get the person to read this book. How this can best be achieved will depend on the exact circumstances and may require considerable sensitivity on your part. Keep in mind that binge eating problems are associated with much shame and self-recrimination, so being "found out" can come as a considerable shock.

If the problem is in the open, the issue may be how you can

help. This will depend on whether your relative or friend wants to change. If ambivalence is a problem, you might help him or her review the section "Why Change?" at the beginning of Part II. On the other hand, if he or she already has a desire to change, you might together review the various options to decide which is best. If the decision is to seek professional treatment, then you can help by facilitating this. And once a therapist has been identified, it may well be appropriate to find out what role, if any, you should take. I must stress, however, that you should avoid becoming overinvolved. Sometimes the most caring thing that you can do is to be there in the background and make yourself available when needed.

If the decision is to use the self-help program, then a backseat role certainly is best. You should familiarize yourself with the program so that you know what it involves, but it will be up to your relative or friend to decide exactly how you can be of most help. Remember, the program involves the person's acting as his or her own therapist. You may be left uninvolved except as someone to provide support or advice at difficult times. This can be a demanding part to play. You may feel tempted to intervene when you should not, or you could be asked to help at an inconvenient time.

It is not uncommon for people tackling their binge eating problem to feel discouraged, even hopeless, at times. They may feel that they will never overcome the problem. If they share such feelings with you, help them review their progress in a balanced way (the review checklists and summary sheets can help), and make sure that all achievements (however trivial they might seem) are highlighted since they often get neglected. Point out all signs of progress and provide as much encouragement as you can.

One other point worth making is that you may feel that the program is too simple to work. If this is your view, it is important to remember that the program is based on what is undoubtedly the most effective treatment available (see Chapter 8). Try not to undermine the program. Instead, suspend your misgivings and support your relative or friend in using the program. In this way you will increase his or her chances of recovery.

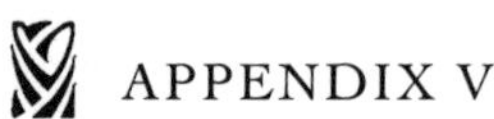

APPENDIX V

A Note for Therapists

AS A THERAPIST HELPING SOMEONE with a binge eating problem, you can take one of two roles with respect to the self-help program in this book (see Part II). You can directly help the person follow the program ("guided self-help"), or you can provide a completely different form of therapy while at the same time supporting his or her use of the program. In the latter case you may decide to have little or no direct involvement with its use. But even with this approach we suggest that you familiarize yourself with the program in case it clashes in any way with the help that you are providing.

Research by Dr. Peter Cooper and colleagues in Cambridge (UK) suggests that guided self-help is a particularly potent way of helping those with binge eating problems. It is certainly an excellent first step in a stepped-care program (see Chapter 8). It involves having the person with the binge eating problem follow the program supported by regular therapy sessions with you. These can be quite brief (less than 30 minutes long) and need not be scheduled every week. Since the program involves the person becoming his or her own therapist, your role differs from that in some more conventional forms of therapy. In guided self-help you act as a facilitator whose primary role is to monitor progress, provide encouragement, and, at times of difficulty, help identify problems and potential solutions. To do this, you need to be thoroughly familiar with the program.

An important aspect of the therapist's role in guided self-help is to keep the person motivated. Reviewing the monitoring records at the beginning of each session is a good way to achieve this since it provides a means of identifying and highlighting progress. Another key task is to ensure that the person moves through the program at an appropriate rate. Some want to go too fast; others want to go too slow. The sections "When to Move On" provide clear guidelines for when it is appropriate to progress from one step to another. A third role is to keep the person focused on the goals of the program—normalizing eating as opposed to attempting to lose weight (see Appendix II). However, you must always maintain a backseat role. The person with the binge eating problem must remain in charge and be the primary source of change.

There is one other way that this book can be helpful. Since it provides sound information and advice, it can be used to supplement more conventional approaches to the treatment of the eating problem. For example, it can be used as an adjunct to conventional cognitive-behavioral therapy or as a component of an inpatient program.

If this book belongs to a colleague or to your client, and you are interested in examining it in greater detail, the publisher is offering a limited number of examination copies of *Overcoming Binge Eating* to health care providers. Call The Guilford Press toll-free at 1-800-365-7006 to request your copy, which may be examined for 30 days with no obligation to purchase. (For examination copies in the United Kingdom, call The Guilford Press at 01 273 207 411.) Please also see the following two pages—they describe two methods for making this volume readily available to your clients.

Quantity Discounts and a Special Service for Recommending *Overcoming Binge Eating*

To the Health Care Professional:

Here are two convenient methods for ordering *Overcoming Binge Eating*.

❶ Quantity Discounts

For multiple copies of *Overcoming Binge Eating,* calculate the following discount rates against the original list price to get the *unit discount price*. Then simply multiply the discount price times the quantity you are ordering. Add 5% of your total order for shipping.

QUANTITY	LIST PRICE	DISCOUNT	PRICE PER BOOK
1 book	$15.95	---	$15.95
2–12 books		20% off list price	$12.76
13–24 books		30% off list price	$11.17
25+		33% off list price	$10.69

To order, please call toll-free 1-800-365-7006

❷ PRIORITY ORDER FORMS

Or, when recommending the book, you may have individuals order directly from Guilford—simply photocopy the Priority Order Form on the next page. Priority Order Forms are given immediate attention.

We also assure confidentiality. Customers who use these order forms will be excluded from the Guilford mailing list and will receive no further correspondence.

We suggest that you also photocopy the order form for future use.

Please note: This form is for U.S. and Canadian orders only. Prices slightly different in the UK. For information, call Psychology Press, UK, at (01273) 207 411.

PHOTOCOPY FOR PERSONAL USE

PRIORITY ORDER FORM

Send to: **Guilford Publications, Inc., Dept.** SELF
72 Spring Street, New York, NY 10012

CALL TOLL-FREE 1-800-365-7006
Mon.–Fri. , 9am–5pm EST
Or **FAX 212-966-6708**

(Be sure to tell the representative you are ordering from our Priority Order Form.)

NAME

ADDRESS

CITY STATE ZIP

DAYTIME PHONE NO.

Method of Payment

☐ Check or money order enclosed.

Please bill my ☐ VISA ☐ MasterCard ☐ AmEx

ACCT. # ☐☐☐☐ ☐☐☐☐ ☐☐☐☐ ☐☐☐☐

Expiration Date: MONTH ☐☐ YEAR ☐☐

SIGNATURE

(required for all credit card orders)

Name of recommending professional:

Please Ship:

Qty.		Cat. #	Amount
1	Overcoming Binge Eating	2179	$15.95
		*Shipping	
		In NY and PA, add sales tax. In Canada, add GST	
		TOTAL	

*Shipping (Via Priority Mail—1 to 2 week delivery): In U.S., add $4.00; in Canada, add US $7.50.

PRIORITY ORDER For office use only
Note: Operator—set up as account type IT—Mail No—Rush Order
SHIP VIA FC

Further Reading

There is only one professional book devoted to the subject of binge eating, and it addresses all the topics covered in this book:

Fairburn, C. G., & Wilson, G. T. (Eds.). (1993). *Binge eating: Nature, assessment, and treatment*. New York: Guilford Press.

For information on eating disorders and obesity in general, the following comprehensive book is recommended:

Brownell, K. D., & Fairburn, C. G. (Eds.). (1995). *Eating disorders and obesity: A comprehensive handbook*. New York: Guilford Press.

Both books can be obtained by writing to Guilford Publications, Inc., Department C, 72 Spring St., New York NY 10012 or by calling toll-free 800-365-7006.

Sources of further information of relevance to each chapter are listed below. The citations refer either to original sources or to good review articles. They are not exhaustive.

PREFACE

Evidence that the mass media are a major source of information on eating disorders:

Murray, S., Touyz, S., & Beumont, P. J. V. (1990). Knowledge about eating disorders in the community. *International Journal of Eating Disorders 9*, 87–93.

Evidence that most cases of bulimia nervosa are not in treatment:

Fairburn, C. G., & Cooper, P. J. (1982). Self-induced vomiting and bulimia nervosa: An undetected problem. *British Medical Journal, 284,* 1153–1155.

Welch, S. L., & Fairburn, C. G. (1994). Sexual abuse and bulimia nervosa: Three integrated case-control comparisons. *American Journal of Psychiatry 151,* 402–407.

Whitaker, A., Johnson, J., Shaffer, D., Rapoport, J. L., Kalikow, K., Walsh, B. T., Davies, M., Braiman S., & Dolinsky, A. (1990). Uncommon troubles among young people: Prevalence estimates of selected psychiatric disorders in a nonreferred adolescent population. *Archives of General Psychiatry 47,* 487–496.

PART I

Chapter 1

Lay use of the term *binge*:

Fairburn, C. G., Beglin, S. J. (1992). What is meant by the term "binge"? *American Journal of Psychiatry 149,* 123–124.

Technical definition of a binge:

American Psychiatric Association (1994). *Diagnostic and statistical manual of mental disorders, fourth edition.* Washington, D.C.: American Psychiatric Association.

Fairburn, C. G., & Wilson, G. T. (1993). Binge eating: Definition and classification. In C. G. Fairburn & G. T. Wilson (Eds.), *Binge eating: Nature, assessment and treatment.* New York: Guilford Press.

A detailed analysis of the psychological processes underlying binge eating:

Polivy, J., & Herman, C. P. (1993). Binge eating: Psychological mechanisms. In C. G. Fairburn & G. T. Wilson (Eds.), *Binge eating: Nature, assessment and treatment.* New York: Guilford Press.

Characteristics of binge eating in bulimia nervosa:

Walsh, B. T. (1993). Binge eating in bulimia nervosa. In C. G. Fairburn & G. T. Wilson (Eds.), *Binge eating: Nature, assessment and treatment.* New York: Guilford Press.

Frequency of binge eating in bulimia nervosa:

Wilson, G. T. & Eldredge, K. L. (1991). Frequency of binge eating in bulimic patients: Diagnostic validity. *International Journal of Eating Disorders 10,* 557–561.

The myth of carbohydrate craving:

Walsh, B. T. (1993). Binge eating in bulimia nervosa. In C. G. Fairburn & G. T. Wilson (Eds.), *Binge eating: Nature, assessment and treatment.* New York: Guilford Press.

The size of binges:

Walsh, B. T. (1993). Binge eating in bulimia nervosa. In C. G. Fairburn & G. T. Wilson (Eds.), *Binge eating: Nature, assessment and treatment.* New York: Guilford Press.

The Eating Disorder Examination:

Fairburn, C. G., & Cooper, Z. (1993). The Eating Disorder Examination (12th edition). In C. G. Fairburn & G. T. Wilson (Eds.), *Binge eating: Nature, assessment and treatment.* New York: Guilford Press.

The cost of binge eating:

Johnson, C. L., Stuckey, M. K., Lewis, L. D., & Schwartz, D. M. (1983). A survey of 509 cases of self-reported bulimia. In P. L. Darby, P. E. Garfinkel, D. M. Garner, & D. V. Coscina (Eds.), *Anorexia nervosa: Recent developments in research.* New York: Alan Liss.

Binge eating in anorexia nervosa:

Garner, D. M. (1993). Binge eating in anorexia nervosa. In C. G. Fairburn & G. T. Wilson (Eds.), *Binge eating: Nature, assessment and treatment.* New York: Guilford Press.

Binge eating in obesity.

Marcus, M. D. (1993). Binge eating in obesity. In C. G. Fairburn & G. T. Wilson (Eds.), *Binge eating: Nature, assessment and treatment.* New York: Guilford Press.

Eating in binge eating disorder:

Yanovski, S. Z., Leet, M., Yanovski, J. A., et al. (1992). Food intake and selection of obese women with binge eating disorder. *American Journal of Clinical Nutrition 56,* 975–980.

Rossiter, E. M., Agras, W. S., Telch C. F., & Bruce, B. (1992).

The eating patterns of non-purging bulimic subjects. *International Journal of Eating Disorders 11,* 111–120.

Goldfein, J. A., Walsh, B. T., LaChaussee, J. L., Kissileff, H. R., & Devlin, M. J. (1993). Eating behavior in binge eating disorder. *International Journal of Eating Disorders 14,* 427–431.

Yanovski, S. Z., & Sebring, N. G. (1994). Recorded food intake of obese women with binge eating disorder before and after weight loss. *International Journal of Eating Disorders 15,* 135–150.

Chapter 2

The classification of eating problems:

Garfinkel, P. E. (1995). Classification and diagnosis of eating disorders. In K. D. Brownell & C. G. Fairburn (Eds.), *Eating disorders and obesity: A comprehensive handbook.* New York: Guilford Press.

Fairburn, C. G. & Walsh, B. T. (1995). Atypical eating disorders. In K. D. Brownell & C. G. Fairburn (Eds.), *Eating disorders and obesity: A comprehensive handbook.* New York: Guilford Press.

Diagnostic criteria for bulimia nervosa:

American Psychiatric Association (1994). *Diagnostic and statistical manual of mental disorders, fourth edition.* Washington, D.C.: American Psychiatric Association.

Diagnostic criteria for binge eating disorder:

American Psychiatric Association (1994). *Diagnostic and statistical manual of mental disorders, fourth edition.* Washington, D.C.: American Psychiatric Association.

Controversial status of binge eating disorder:

Fairburn, C. G., Welch, S. L., & Hay, P. J. (1993). The classification of recurrent overeating: The "binge eating disorder" proposal. *International Journal of Eating Disorders 13,* 155–159.

Fichter, M. M., Quadflieg, N. & Brandl, B. (1993). Recurrent overeating: An empirical comparison of binge eating disorder, bulimia nervosa, and obesity. *International Journal of Eating Disorders 14,* 1–16.

Argument for binge eating disorder:

Devlin, M. J., Walsh, B. T., Spitzer, R. L., & Hasin, D. (1992). Is there another binge eating disorder?: A review of the literature on overeating in the absence of bulimia. *International Journal of Eating Disorders 11,* 333–340.

Spitzer, R. L., Devlin, M. J., Walsh, B. T., Hasin, D., Wing, R. R., Marcus, M. D., Stunkard, A., Wadden, T. A., Yanovski, S., Agras, W. S., Mitchell, J. & Nonas, C. (1992). Binge eating disorder: A multisite field trial for the diagnostic criteria. *International Journal of Eating Disorders 11,* 191–203.

Spitzer, R. L., Yanovski, S., Wadden, T., Wing, R., Marcus, M. D., Stunkard, A., Devlin, M., Mitchell, J., Hasin, D. & Horne, R. L. (1993). Binge eating disorder: Its further validation in a multisite study. *International Journal of Eating Disorders 13,* 137–153.

Diagnostic criteria for anorexia nervosa:

American Psychiatric Association (1994). *Diagnostic and statistical manual of mental disorders, fourth edition.* Washington, D.C.: American Psychiatric Association.

Binge eating in anorexia nervosa:

Garner, D. M. (1993). Binge eating in anorexia nervosa. In C. G. Fairburn & G. T. Wilson (Eds.), *Binge eating: Nature, assessment and treatment.* New York: Guilford Press.

Chapter 3

Russell's seminal paper on bulimia nervosa:

Russell, G. F. M. (1979). Bulimia nervosa: An ominous variant of anorexia nervosa. *Psychological Medicine 9,* 429–448.

The Cosmopolitan study:

Fairburn, C. G., & Cooper, P. J. (1982). Self-induced vomiting and bulimia nervosa: An undetected problem. *British Medical Journal 284,* 1153–1155.

The Chicago study:

Johnson, C. L., Stuckey, M. K., Lewis, L. D., & Schwartz, D. M. (1983). A survey of 509 cases of self-reported bulimia. In P.L. Darby, P.E. Garfinkel, D.M. Garner, & D.V. Coscina (Eds.), *Anorexia nervosa: Recent developments in research.* New York: Alan Liss.

The Cornell Study:

Halmi, K. A., Falk, J. R., & Schwartz, E. (1981). Binge-eating and vomiting: A survey of a college population. *Psychological Medicine 11,* 697–706.

The detection of bulimia nervosa:

Welch, S. L., & Fairburn, C. G. (1994). Sexual abuse and bulimia nervosa: Three integrated case-control comparisons. *American Journal of Psychiatry 151,* 402–407.

Whitaker, A., Johnson, J., Shaffer, D., Rapoport, J. L., Kalikow, K., Walsh, B. T., Davies, M., Braiman S., & Dolinsky, A. (1990). Uncommon troubles among young people: Prevalence estimates of selected psychiatric disorders in a nonreferred adolescent population. *Archives of General Psychiatry 47,* 487–496.

Studies of the distribution of binge eating problems:

Fairburn, C. G., & Beglin, S. J. (1990). Studies of the epidemiology of bulimia nervosa. *American Journal of Psychiatry 147,* 401–408.

Hoek, H. W. (1995). The distribution of eating disorders. In K. D. Brownell & C. G. Fairburn (Eds.), *Eating disorders and obesity: A comprehensive handbook.* New York: Guilford Press.

The prevalence of bulimia nervosa among men:

Fairburn, C. G., & Cooper, P. J. (1984). Binge eating, self-induced vomiting and laxative abuse: A community study. *Psychological Medicine 14,* 401–410.

Bushnell, J. A., Wells, J. E., Hornblow, A. R., Oakley-Browne, M. A., & Joyce, P. (1990). Prevalence of three bulimia syndromes in the general population. *Psychological Medicine 20,* 671–680.

Distribution of binge eating disorder:

Spitzer, R. L., Devlin, M. J., Walsh, B. T., Hasin, D., Wing, R. R., Marcus, M. D., Stunkard, A., Wadden, T. A., Yanovski, S., Agras, W. S., Mitchell, J. & Nonas, C. (1992). Binge eating disorder: A multisite field trial for the diagnostic criteria. *International Journal of Eating Disorders 11,* 191–203.

Spitzer, R. L., Yanovski, S., Wadden, T., Wing, R., Marcus, M. D., Stunkard, A., Devlin, M., Mitchell, J., Hasin, D. & Horne, R. L. (1993). Binge eating disorder: Its further validation in a multisite study. *International Journal of Eating Disorders 13,* 137–153.

Binge eating problems in obesity:

Marcus, M. D. (1993). Binge eating in obesity. In C. G. Fairburn & G. T. Wilson (Eds.), *Binge eating: Nature, assessment and treatment.* New York: Guilford Press.

Wilson, G. T., Nonas, C. A., & Rosenblum, G. D. (1993). Assessment of binge eating in obese patients. *International Journal of Eating Disorders 13,* 25–33.

Binge eating problems among those with diabetes mellitus:

Peveler, R. C. (1995). Eating disorders and diabetes. In K. D. Brownell & C. G. Fairburn (Eds.), *Eating disorders and obesity: A comprehensive handbook.* New York: Guilford Press.

Are binge eating problems becoming more common?:

New Zealand—Bushnell, J. A., Wells, J. E., Hornblow, A. R., Oakley-Browne, M. A., & Joyce, P. (1990). Prevalence of three bulimia syndromes in the general population. *Psychological Medicine 20,* 671–680.

United States—Kendler, K. S., MacLean, C., Neale, M., Kessler, R., Heath, A., & Eaves, L. (1991). The genetic epidemiology of bulimia nervosa. *American Journal of Psychiatry 148,* 1627–1637.

Canada—Garner, D. M., Fairburn, C. G. (1988). Relationship between anorexia nervosa and bulimia nervosa: Diagnostic implications. In D. M. Garner and P. E. Garfinkel (Eds.), *Diagnostic issues in anorexia nervosa and bulimia nervosa.* New York: Brunner/Mazel.

New Zealand—Hall, A. & Hay, P. J. (1991). Eating disorder patient referrals from a population region 1977–1986. *Psychological Medicine 21,* 697–701.

United Kingdom—Lacey, J. H. (1992). The treatment demand for bulimia: A catchment area report of referral rates and demography. *Psychiatric Bulletin 16,* 203–205.

Chapter 4

Dieting and binge eating:

Polivy, J. & Herman, C. P. (1993). Binge eating: Psychological mechanisms. In C. G. Fairburn & G. T. Wilson (Eds.), *Binge eating: Nature, assessment and treatment.* New York: Guilford Press.

Overeating in binge eating disorder:

Yanovski, S. Z., Leet, M., Yanovski, J. A., et al. (1992). Food intake and selection of obese women with binge eating disorder. *American Journal of Clinical Nutrition 56,* 975–980.

Rossiter, E. M., Agras, W. S., Telch C. F., & Bruce, B. (1992). The eating patterns of non-purging bulimic subjects. *International Journal of Eating Disorders 11,* 111–120.

Goldfein, J. A., Walsh, B. T., LaChaussee, J. L., Kissileff, H. R., &

Devlin, M. J. (1993). Eating behavior in binge eating disorder. *International Journal of Eating Disorders 14,* 427–431.

Yanovski, S. Z., & Sebring, N. G. (1994). Recorded food intake of obese women with binge eating disorder before and after weight loss. *International Journal of Eating Disorders 15,* 135–150.

Does self-induced vomiting work?:

Kaye, W. H., Weltzin, T. E., Hsu, L. K. G., McConaha, C. W., & Bolton, B. (1993). Amount of calories retained after binge eating and vomiting. *American Journal of Psychiatry 150,* 969–971.

Vomiting encourages binge eating:

Rosen, J. C., & Leitenberg, H. (1988). The anxiety model of bulimia nervosa and treatment with exposure plus response prevention. In K. M. Pirke, W. Vandereycken, & D. Ploog (Eds.), *The psychobiology of bulimia nervosa* (146–151). Berlin: Springer-Verlag.

Overexercising as a feature of eating disorders:

Beumont, P. J. V., Arthur, B., Russell, J. D., & Touyz, S. W. (1994). Excessive physical activity in dieting disorder patients. *International Journal of Eating Disorders 15,* 21– 36.

"Normative discontent":

Rodin, J., Silberstein L., & Striegel-Moore R. (1984). Women and weight: A normative discontent. In T. B. Sonderegger (Ed.), *Nebraska symposium on motivation.* Lincoln: University of Nebraska Press.

Depressive and anxiety symptoms in bulimia nervosa:

Cooper, P. J. (1995). Eating disorders and their relationship to mood and anxiety disorders. In K. D. Brownell & C. G. Fairburn (Eds.), *Eating disorders and obesity: A comprehensive handbook.* New York: Guilford Press.

Depressive and anxiety symptoms in binge eating disorder:

Marcus, M. D. (1993). Binge eating in obesity. In C. G. Fairburn & G. T. Wilson (Eds.), *Binge eating: Nature, assessment and treatment.* New York: Guilford Press.

Childrearing of mothers with bulimia nervosa:

Stein, A. (1995). Eating disorders and childrearing. In K. D. Brownell & C. G. Fairburn (Eds.), *Eating disorders and obesity: A comprehensive handbook.* New York: Guilford Press.

Personality and binge eating problems:

Wonderlich, S. A. (1995). Personality and eating disorders. In K. D. Brownell & C. G. Fairburn (Eds.), *Eating disorders and obesity: A comprehensive handbook.* New York: Guilford Press.

The "multi-impulsive" personality:

Lacey, J. H., & Evans, C. D. H. (1986). The impulsivist: A multi-impulsive personality disorder. *British Journal of Addiction 81,* 641–649.

Personality disorder and treatment outcome:

Johnson, C., Tobin, D., & Dennis, A. B. (1990). Differences in treatment outcome between borderline and nonborderline bulimics at one-year follow-up. *International Journal of Eating Disorders 9,* 617–628.

Rossiter, E. M., Agras, W. S., Telch, C. F., & Schneider, J. A. (1993). Cluster B personality disorder characteristics predict outcome in the treatment of bulimia nervosa. *International Journal of Eating Disorders 13,* 349–358.

Wonderlich, S. A., Fullerton, D., Swift W. J., & Klein M. H. (1994). Five-year outcome from eating disorders: Relevance of personality disorders. *International Journal of Eating Disorders 15,* 233–244.

Pregnancy and eating disorders:

Lacey, J. H., & Smith, G. (1987). Bulimia nervosa: The impact of pregnancy on mother and baby. *British Journal of Psychiatry 150,* 777–781.

Fairburn, C. G., Stein, A., Jones, R. (1992). Eating habits and eating disorders during pregnancy. *Psychosomatic Medicine 5,* 665–672.

Franko, D. L. & Walton B. F. (1993). Pregancy and eating disorders: A review and clinical implications. *International Journal of Eating Disorders 13,* 41–48.

Chapter 5

Physical problems associated with binge eating and bulimia nervosa:

Mitchell, J. E. (1995). Medical complications of bulimia nervosa. In K. D. Brownell & C. G. Fairburn (Eds.), *Eating disorders and obesity: A comprehensive handbook.* New York: Guilford Press.

Kaplan, A. S. & Garfinkel P. E. (Eds.). (1993). *Medical issues and the eating disorders: The interface.* New York: Brunner/Mazel.

"Natural weight" and bulimia nervosa:

Russell, G. F. M. (1988). The diagnostic formulation in bulimia nervosa. In D. M. Garner and P. E. Garfinkel (Eds.), *Diagnostic issues in anorexia nervosa and bulimia nervosa*. New York: Brunner/Mazel.

Effects of treatment on weight:

Fairburn, C. G., Jones, R., Peveler, R. C., Hope, R. A., O'Connor, M. E. (1993). Psychotherapy and bulimia nervosa: The longer-term effects of interpersonal psychotherapy, behaviour therapy and cognitive behaviour therapy. *Archives of General Psychiatry 50,* 419–428.

Weight cycling (yo-yo dieting):

Wing, R. R. (1992). Weight cycling in humans: A review of the literature. *Annals of Behavioral Medicine 14,* 113–119.

Weight cycling and health:

Lissner L., Odell, P. M., D'Agostino, R. D., Stokes, J., Kreger, B. E., Belanger, A. J., & Brownell, K. D. (1991). Variability of body weight and health outcomes in the Framingham population. *New England Journal of Medicine 324,* 1839–1844.

Dieting and the mechanisms that control eating:

Blundell, J. E. & Hill A. J. (1993). Binge eating: Psychobiological mechanisms. In C. G. Fairburn & G. T. Wilson (Eds.), *Binge eating: Nature, assessment and treatment*. New York: Guilford Press.

Dieting and brain neurotransmitters:

Cowen, P. J., Anderson, I. M., & Fairburn, C. G. (1992). Neurochemical effects of dieting: Relevance to changes in eating and affective disorder. In G. H. Anderson & S. H. Kennedy (Eds.), *The biology of feast and famine: Relevance to eating disorders*. New York: Academic Press.

Ipecac abuse:

Greenfield, D., Mickley, D., Quinlan, D. M., & Roloff, P. (1993). Ipecac abuse in a sample of eating disordered outpatients. *International Journal of Eating Disorders 13,* 411–414.

Effects on fertility and pregnancy:

Goldbloom, D. S. (1993). Menstrual and reproductive function in the eating disorders. In A. S. Kaplan & P. E. Garfinkel (Eds.), *Medical issues and the eating disorders: The interface*. New York: Brunner/Mazel.

Miscarriage rate in bulimia nervosa:

Mitchell, J. E., Seim, H. C., Glotter, D., Soll, E. A., Pyle, R. L. (1991). A retrospective study of pregnancy in bulimia nervosa. *International Journal of Eating Disorders 10,* 209–214.

Chapter 6

Identifying causes: A two-part problem:

Cooper, Z. (1995). The development and maintenance of eating disorders. In K. D. Brownell & C. G. Fairburn (Eds.), *Eating disorders and obesity: A comprehensive handbook.* New York: Guilford Press.

Social and developmental factors:

Vandereycken, W. & Hoek, H. W. (1993). Are eating disorders culture-bound syndromes? In K. A. Halmi (Ed.), *Psychobiology and treatment of anorexia nervosa and bulimia nervosa.* Washington, D.C.: American Psychiatric Press.

Dolan, B. (1991). Cross-cultural aspects of anorexia nervosa and bulimia: A review. *International Journal of Eating Disorders 10,* 67–78.

Striegel-Moore, R. H. (1993). Etiology of binge eating: A developmental perspective. In C. G. Fairburn & G. T. Wilson (Eds.), *Binge eating: Nature, assessment and treatment.* New York: Guilford Press.

Levine M. P. & Smolak L. (1992). Toward a model of the developmental psychopathology of eating disorders: The example of early adolescence. In J. H. Crowther, D. L. Tennenbaum, S. E. Hobfoll, & M. A. P. Stephens (Eds.), *The etiology of bulimia nervosa: The individual and familial context.* Washington, D.C.: Hemisphere.

Eating disorders and men:

Andersen, A. E. (Ed.). (1990). *Males with eating disorders.* New York: Brunner/Mazel.

Genetics of weight and obesity:

Grilo C. M. & Pogue-Geile M. F. (1991). The nature of environmental influences on weight and obesity: A behavior genetic analysis. *Psychological Bulletin 110,* 520–537.

Eating problems and disorders within the family:

Strober, M. (1995). Family-genetic perspectives on anorexia nervosa and bulimia nervosa. In K. D. Brownell & C. G. Fairburn (Eds.), *Eating disorders and obesity: A comprehensive handbook.* New York: Guilford Press.

Kendler, K. S., MacLean, C., Neale, M., Kessler, R., Heath, A., & Eaves, L. (1991). The genetic epidemiology of bulimia nervosa. *American Journal of Psychiatry 148,* 1627–1637.

Wonderlich, S. A. (1992). Relationship of family and personality factors in bulimia. In J. H. Crowther, D. L. Tennenbaum, S. E. Hobfoll, & M. A. P. Stephens (Eds.), *The etiology of bulimia nervosa: The individual and familial context.* Washington, D.C.: Hemisphere.

Vandereycken, W. (1995). The families of patients with an eating disorder. In K. D. Brownell & C. G. Fairburn (Eds.), *Eating disorders and obesity: A comprehensive handbook.* New York: Guilford Press.

Sexual abuse and eating disorders:

Palmer, R. L. (1995). Sexual abuse and eating disorders. In K. D. Brownell & C. G. Fairburn (Eds.), *Eating disorders and obesity: A comprehensive handbook.* New York: Guilford Press.

Pope, H. G. & Hudson, J. I. (1992). Is childhood sexual abuse a risk factor for bulimia nervosa? *American Journal of Psychiatry 149,* 455–463.

Welch, S. L. & Fairburn, C. G. (1994). Sexual abuse and bulimia nervosa: Three integrated case-control comparisons. *American Journal of Psychiatry 151,* 402–407.

Personality and eating disorders:

Wonderlich, S. A. (1995). Personality and eating disorders. In K. D. Brownell & C. G. Fairburn (Eds.), *Eating disorders and obesity: A comprehensive handbook.* New York: Guilford Press.

Wonderlich, S. A. (1992). Relationship of family and personality factors in bulimia. In J. H. Crowther, D. L. Tennenbaum, S. E. Hobfoll & M. A. P. Stephens (Eds.), *The etiology of bulimia nervosa: The individual and familial context.* Washington, D.C.: Hemisphere.

Johnson, C., Wonderlich, S. (1992). Personality characteristics as a risk factor in the development of eating disorders. In J. H. Crowther, D. L. Tennenbaum, S. E. Hobfoll, & M. A. P. Stephens (Eds.), *The etiology of bulimia nervosa: The individual and familial context.* Washington, D.C.: Hemisphere.

Strober, M. (1991). Disorders of the self in anorexia nervosa: An organismic-developmental paradigm. In C. Johnson (Ed.), *Psychodynamic treatment of anorexia nervosa and bulimia.* New York: Guilford Press.

Dieting as a risk factor:

Heatherton, T. F., & Polivy J. (1992). Chronic dieting and eating disorders: A spiral model. In J. H. Crowther, D. L. Tennenbaum, S. E. Hobfoll & M. A. P. Stephens, (Eds.), *The etiology of bulimia nervosa: The individual and familial context*. Washington, D.C.: Hemisphere.

Patton, G. C., Johnson-Sabine, E., Wood, K., Mann, A. H., & Wakeling, A. (1990). Abnormal eating attitudes in London schoolgirls—A prospective epidemiological study: outcome at twelve month follow-up. *Psychological Medicine 20,* 383–394.

Chapter 7

Binge eating and addiction:

Wilson, G. T. (1993). Binge eating and addictive disorders. In C. G. Fairburn & G. T. Wilson (Eds.), *Binge eating: Nature, assessment and treatment*. New York: Guilford Press.

Bemis, K. M. (1985). "Abstinence" and "nonabstinence" models for the treatment of bulimia. *International Journal of Eating Disorders 4,* 407–437.

Vandereycken, W. (1990). The addiction model in eating disorders: Some critical remarks and a selected bibliography. *International Journal of Eating Disorders 9,* 95–101.

Chapter 8

The research on the treatment of bulimia nervosa:

Fairburn, C. G., Agras, W. S., & Wilson, G. T. (1992). The research on the treatment of bulimia nervosa: Practical and theoretical implications. In G. H. Anderson & S. H. Kennedy (Eds.), *The biology of feast and famine: Relevance to eating disorders*. San Diego: Academic Press.

The need for treatment to produce lasting change:

Keller, M. B., Herzog, D. B., Lavori, I. S., Bradburn, E. M., & Mahoney, E. M. (1992). The naturalistic history of bulimia nervosa: Extraordinarily high rates of chronicity, relapse, recurrence, and psychosocial morbidity. *International Journal of Eating Disorders 12,* 1–10.

Drug treatment of eating disorders:

Walsh, B. T. (1995). Pharmacotherapy of eating disorders. In K. D.

Brownell & C. G. Fairburn (Eds.), *Eating disorders and obesity: A comprehensive handbook.* New York: Guilford Press.

The "New Hope" book:

Pope, H. G., & Hudson, J. I. (1984). *New hope for binge eaters.* New York: Harper & Row.

Difficulty recruiting patients for drug trials:

Leitenberg, H., Rosen, J. C., Wolf, J., Vara, L. S., Detzer, M. J., & Srebnik, D. (1994). Comparison of cognitive-behavior therapy and desipramine in the treatment of bulimia nervosa. *Behaviour Research and Therapy 32,* 37–45.

Effectiveness of antidepressants in the longer-term:

Walsh, B. T., Hadigan, B. A., Devlin, M. J., Gladis, M., & Roose, S. P. (1991). Long-term outcome of antidepressant treatment for bulimia nervosa. *American Journal of Psychiatry 148,* 1206–1212.

Lack of effect of antidepressant drugs on dietary restriction:

Rossiter, E. M., Agras, W. S., Losch, M., & Telch, C. F. (1988). Dietary restraint of bulimic subjects following cognitive-behavioral or pharmacological treatment. *Behaviour Research and Therapy 26,* 495–498.

Cognitive-behavioral therapy for binge eating and bulimia nervosa:

Fairburn, C. G. (1981). A cognitive behavioural approach to the treatment of bulimia. *Psychological Medicine 11,* 707–711.

Wilson, G. T., & Fairburn, C. G. (1993). Cognitive treatments for eating disorders. *Journal of Consulting and Clinical Psychology 61,* 261–269.

Fairburn, C. G., Marcus, M. D., & Wilson, G. T. (1993). Cognitive behaviour therapy for binge eating and bulimia nervosa: A treatment manual. In C. G. Fairburn & G. T. Wilson (Eds.), *Binge eating: Nature, assessment and treatment.* New York: Guilford Press.

The Oxford study of the longer-term effects of cognitive-behavioral therapy:

Fairburn, C. G., Jones, R., Peveler, R. C., Hope, R. A., & O'Connor, M. E. (1993). Psychotherapy and bulimia nervosa: the longer-term effects of interpersonal psychotherapy, behaviour therapy and cognitive behaviour therapy. *Archives of General Psychiatry 50,* 419–428.

Cognitive-behavioral therapy for binge eating disorder:

Telch, C. F., Agras, W. S., Rossiter, E. M., Wilfley, D., & Kenardy, J. (1990). Group cognitive-behavioral treatment for the non-purging bulimic: an initial evaluation. *Journal of Consulting and Clinical Psychology 58,* 629–635.

Smith, D. E., Marcus, M. D., & Kaye, W. (1992). Cognitive-behavioral treatment of obese binge eaters. *International Journal of Eating Disorders 12,* 257–262.

Wilfley, D. E., Agras, W. S., Telch, C. F., Rossiter, E.M., Schneider, J. A., Cole, A. G., Sifford, L., & Raeburn, S. D. (1993). Group cognitive-behavioral therapy and group interpersonal psychotherapy for the nonpurging bulimic individual: A controlled comparison. *Journal of Consulting and Clinical Psychology 61,* 296–305.

Behavior therapy for binge eating problems:

Rosen, J. C., & Leitenberg, H. (1988). The anxiety model of bulimia nervosa and treatment with exposure plus response prevention. In K. M. Pirke, W. Vandereycken, & D. Ploog (Eds.), *The psychobiology of bulimia nervosa.* Berlin: Springer-Verlag.

Agras, W. S., Schneider, J. A., Arnow, B., Raeburn, S. D., & Telch, C. F. (1989). Cognitive-behavioral and response-prevention treatments for bulimia nervosa. *Journal of Consulting and Clinical Psychology 57,* 215–221.

Leitenberg, H., Rosen, J. C., Gross, J., Nudelman, S., & Vara, L. S. (1988). Exposure plus response-prevention treatment of bulimia nervosa. *Journal of Consulting and Clinical Psychology 56,* 535–541.

Wilson, G. T., Eldredge, K. L., Smith, D., & Niles, B. (1991). Cognitive-behavioral treatment with and without response prevention for bulimia. *Behaviour Research and Therapy 29,* 575–583.

Fairburn, C. G., Jones, R., Peveler, R. C., Hope, R. A., & O'-Connor, M. E. (1993). Psychotherapy and bulimia nervosa: the longer-term effects of interpersonal psychotherapy, behaviour therapy and cognitive behaviour therapy. *Archives of General Psychiatry 50,* 419–428.

Psychoeducational treatments:

Olmsted, M. P., & Kaplan, A. S. (1995). Psychoeducation in the treatment of eating disorders. In K. D. Brownell & C. G. Fairburn (Eds.), *Eating disorders and obesity: A comprehensive handbook.* New York: Guilford Press.

Olmsted, M.P., Davis, R., Rockert, W., Irvine, M., Eagle, M., & Garner, D. M. (1991). Efficacy of a brief group psychoeducational intervention for bulimia nervosa. *Behaviour Research and Therapy 29,* 71–83.

Focal psychotherapy:

Fairburn, C. G. (1993). Interpersonal psychotherapy for bulimia nervosa. In G. L. Klerman & M. M. Weissman (Eds.), *New applications of interpersonal psychotherapy.* Washington, D.C.: American Psychiatric Press.

Fairburn, C. G., Jones, R., Peveler, R. C., Hope, R. A., & O'Connor, M. E. (1993). Psychotherapy and bulimia nervosa: the longer-term effects of interpersonal psychotherapy, behaviour therapy and cognitive behaviour therapy. *Archives of General Psychiatry 50,* 419–428.

Wilfley, D. E., Agras, W. S., Telch, C. F., Rossiter, E. M., Schneider, J. A., Cole, A. G., Sifford, L., & Raeburn, S. D. (1993). Group cognitive-behavioral therapy and group interpersonal psychotherapy for the nonpurging bulimic individual: A controlled comparison. *Journal of Consulting and Clinical Psychology 61,* 296–305.

Stepped care and self-help:

Cooper, P.J., Coker, S., & Fleming, C. (1994). Self-help for bulimia nervosa: A preliminary report. *International Journal of Eating Disorders 16,* 401–404.

Fairburn, C. G., & Peveler, R. C. (1990). Bulimia nervosa and a stepped care approach to management. *Gut 31,* 1220–1222.

Fairburn, C. G., Agras, W. S., & Wilson, G. T. (1992). The research on the treatment of bulimia nervosa: Practical and theoretical implications. In G. H. Anderson, & S. H. Kennedy (Eds.), *The biology of feast and famine: Relevance to eating disorders.* San Diego: Academic Press.

Schmidt, U., Tiller, J., & Treasure, J. (1993). Self-treatment of bulimia nervosa: A pilot study. *International Journal of Eating Disorders 13,* 273–277.

Treasure, J., Schmidt, U., Troop, N., Tiller, J., Todd, G., Keilen, M., & Dodge, E. (1994). First step in managing bulimia nervosa: Controlled trial of therapeutic manual. *British Medical Journal 308,* 686–689.

PART II

The cognitive-behavioral treatment on which the program is based:

Fairburn, C. G., Marcus, M. D., & Wilson, G. T. (1993). Cognitive behaviour therapy for binge eating and bulimia nervosa: A treatment manual. In C. G. Fairburn & G. T. Wilson (Eds.),

Binge eating: Nature, assessment and treatment. New York: Guilford Press.

An excellent self-help version of the cognitive-behavioral treatment for bulimia nervosa:

Cooper, P. J. (1995). *Bulimia nervosa and binge eating: A guide to recovery.* London: Robinson.

Dealing with other problems:

Kano, S. (1989). *Making peace with food.* New York: Harper & Row.

Rodin, J. (1992). *Body traps.* New York: William Morrow & Company.

Wolf, N. (1991). *The beauty myth.* New York: Harper & Row.

Orbach, S. (1978). *Fat is a feminist issue.* London: Paddington Press.

Chernin, K. (1985). *The hungry self.* New York: Harper & Row.

Bovey, S. (1989). *Being fat is not a sin.* London: Pandora.

Burns, D. D. (1992). *Feeling good: The new mood therapy.* New York: Avon.

Burns, D. D. (1990). *The feeling good handbook.* New York: Plume.

Russianoff, P. (1991). *When am I going to be happy?* London: Mandarin.

Smith, M. J. (1975). *When I say no, I feel guilty.* New York: Bantam.

Burns, D. D. (1985). *Intimate connections.* New York: Signet.

APPENDICES

Genetics of weight and obesity:

Grilo, C. M., & Pogue-Geile, M. F. (1991). The nature of environmental influences on weight and obesity: A behavior genetic analysis. *Psychological Bulletin 110,* 520–537.

Effectiveness of dietary and behavioral treatments for obesity:

Wilson, G. T. (1994). Behavioral treatment of obesity: Thirty years and counting. *Advances in Behaviour Therapy and Research 16,* 31–75.

Consumer Union. Losing weight. What works. What doesn't. *Consumer Reports,* June 1993.

Healthy eating:

Woteki, C. E., & Thomas, P. R. (1992). *Eat for life: The food and nutrition board's guide to reducing your risk of chronic disease.* Washington, D.C.: National Academy Press.

The LEARN program:

Brownell, K. D. (1993). *The LEARN program for weight control.* Dallas: American Health Publishing Co.

Effectiveness of dietary and behavioral treatments for obesity:

Wilson, G. T. (1994). Behavioral treatment of obesity: Thirty years and counting. *Advances in Behaviour Therapy and Research 16,* 31–75.

Consumer Union. Losing weight. What works. What doesn't. *Consumer Reports,* June 1993.

The concept of a "natural weight":

Polivy, J., & Herman, C. P. (1993). *Breaking the diet habit.* New York: Basic Books.

Index